I happen**d** **upon**
a health club ad with
a particular emphasis
on "total fitness." It
also advertised "No
Dues Till the End of
Summer"! So, no doubt
with mixed motivations,
I discovered myself
opening the door to
an entirely new
experience. . . .

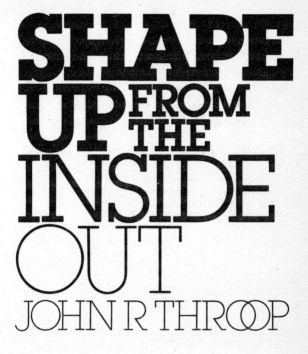

SHAPE UP FROM THE INSIDE OUT

JOHN R THROOP

LIVING BOOKS
Tyndale House Publishers, Inc.
Wheaton, Illinois

To Joe and Dave, who encouraged me;
and for the people of
St. Simon's Episcopal Church,
Arlington Heights, Illinois,
for their prayerful support.

All Scripture quotations are from the
New International Version.

Cover photo credit:
The Image Bank/Janeart, Ltd.

Second printing, July 1986
Library of Congress Catalog Card Number 85-52096
ISBN 0-8423-5899-4
Copyright © 1986 by John R. Throop
Printed in the United States of America

CONTENTS

PREFACE

My wife, Isabel, and I were at a social gathering one afternoon when the same question was asked of me for the thousandth time (or so it seemed): "How did you do it?"

The "it" was my weight loss and physical transformation in the sight of those who had known me as overweight. Pastors live in the public eye to such a degree that some people seem to chart their weight along with other observations. My change was readily noticed. I must admit that I began to grow tired of answering the same question. I liked my new look and simply wanted to get on with enjoying it. But people wanted me to share some practical advice to help them with their own weight problems, and to give them encouragement in other areas of their lives in which they lacked discipline. I finally realized that they were asking for help, not merely being curious about my life history.

Isabel said to me a little later, only half-seriously, "You ought to write a book about it. Then you wouldn't have to answer the question again!'' And the book was born.

Isabel has been the inspiration and moral support behind the writing of this book. Her editing skill also has helped me to write far better than I could have written on my own. Dr. Wendell Hawley at Tyndale House Publishers gave encouragement and guidance as the book took shape. David Neff, editor at *HIS* magazine, ran a short article that was the precursor of this work, and provided many helpful suggestions. The people at St. Simon's Episcopal Church were the greatest encouragement any associate pastor could want. The Rev. Richard E. Lundberg, rector of the parish, shaped my thinking about spiritual dimensions of fitness, and was a great support to me in my discipline. Finally, Dave Mills, Joe Ignoffo, and Maggie Foster, instructors at the Chicago Health Club in Schaumburg, Illinois, at the time I began my journey to fitness, are the authors behind the author. They made the book possible for me to write.

John R. Throop
Shaker Heights, Ohio

INTRODUCTION

For a Christian, getting into shape is as much a spiritual as a physical experience. Because our bodies are intended to be temples of the Holy Spirit, losing weight and becoming fit cannot be considered mere narcissistic self-adoration or obsessive self-concern. Shaping up means nothing less than giving God the honor and adoration due him, because he gave you your body. If we really believe that God took human flesh, that he dwelt fully and completely in Jesus Christ, then we must declare that God loves the human body as much as he does the individual soul. He longs to fill us with his holy and life-giving Spirit, bringing healing to our whole selves.

I tell you that it is not only possible, it is certain that you can become a better steward of the glorious and unique body which God has given you. I testify to you out of my own experience that, in handing your life over to Jesus Christ, he becomes Lord of all that you are, all that you have, *and all that you eat and drink.* Only in asking him to reign over all of your life do you have the remotest possibility of strengthening your will. And only then will you be able to accomplish his purposes in your life.

If you have a weight problem right now, you can become a new person, no matter how much or how little weight you must lose, how good or how bad your physical condition. God desires that you become happy, healthy, and fit.

You must make me a promise as you read this book—actually, two promises: First, I want you to be in prayer as you prepare for the diet and exercise program *you* think you can undertake. Understand *why* you are choosing such a program, and what might hinder you personally from reaching your goal. God will strengthen you to overcome those obstacles. You're asking God to help free you of a subtle and difficult human habit: overeating.

You need to eat. But you probably eat too much and you may eat the wrong things. God wants you to eat right and feel good. Pray that he will transform your unruly will in this area of your life. Admit that you don't have the power to overcome this on your own. Unless you do this honestly, you won't lose a pound.

Second—this may actually be more difficult to accomplish—*don't eat a thing* while you read this book. You'll have to start dealing with your will sometime, and now is as good a time to begin that process as any I know—because it's immediate. Just for good measure, put away those colas and chips or whatever right now. Don't assume that you won't consume! You've got to become aware right now of your desire to eat—and begin to control it.

So you've promised me that, at least while reading

this book, you will fast and pray. That's a good biblical way to begin, a way to honor God from the start, for the change he wants to work in you. Set a time to begin, on whichever diet you choose. Set up an appointment with your doctor. Talk over your new goals with your family and friends. Have them pray for you and even join you in your plan, if they wish. But you're going to have to deal with your own desire to eat. No one else can do it for you.

God can work a change in you. Trust him. He's a great temple builder—and does a nice job of redecorating, too! I know. This book is the story of how he has worked in me. He wants to work his renewing power in you, too.

ONE
SUBSTANTIAL
BEGINNINGS

My heart raced as I walked up to the health club entrance. "What am I doing here?" I thought as I huffed and puffed up the long walk. The sweat poured off of me like the Mississippi River, forming damp spots all over my shirt and suit. "This is crazy! I'm crazy!" I said under my breath—when I could get one.

As I neared the door, I saw a man about my age who had just had his workout. He was muscular, trim, and very tan, just like those models who display the clothes you think *no one* could ever wear. He was wearing those clothes. He had the look of health and well-being. And me? I was 225 pounds of sheer discouragement as I looked at myself. The sweat nearly mingled with tears. "This is impossible!" But something, Someone really, pushed me through the door and led me on; I felt as though I had crossed a boundary which I would leave behind forever.

You must understand that I had been overweight for nearly fourteen years—from about age eleven on.

For someone in his twenties, that's nearly all of recorded history! I really couldn't remember a time when I had been thin, though my parents insist that I was a rail-thin child. Perhaps the onset of adolescence caused certain chemical and hormonal changes in my body which made me more prone to gain weight. I also recall that Mrs. Curtis, our next-door neighbor during one crucial year, made the best fudge, fried foods, and Biloxi black bean soup I'd ever known. She was as wide as she was tall. Her image did not augur well for me.

I also managed to contract pneumonia at the tender age of thirteen, just when those adolescent hormones were most active. I was housebound for six weeks, and out of sheer boredom I began to eat. And eat. And eat. Not vegetables, mind you, nor good, hearty meat dishes, but *pasta*. Any shape, any size, no matter—I craved pasta, with loads of butter and salt. Have you ever seen pictures of cattle at the feeding trough contentedly munching on grain? Well, maybe I wasn't *that* bad. All I know is that I had to wear entirely new and larger clothes when I finally waddled back to school—and I had had a pretty good start on sizes as it was.

I learned in those early years that I like to eat. I was never one of those children who had to be coaxed to finish his plate. I enjoyed all the dishes my mother fixed, and often took seconds. And thirds. My mother, like most mothers, I imagine, was quite pleased to have a child eat well and appreciate her hard work in the kitchen.

I'm from a large, tightly knit family. We moved around quite a bit when I was young, due to my father's work; so, in new communities, we all would stick together. Nonetheless, I sometimes felt lonely and would go into my room and read. When I would read, I would eat. Deep in my mind, then, from an early age, I connected eating with family togetherness, with boredom, and with study. Now, these are three of the most unlikely food partners. But notice that food and living go together for me. For me, to eat is to live, and to live is to eat. It's that simple.

Is that true for you, too? Deep within, I developed a pattern of behaviors revolving around food—its preparation, consumption, and enjoyment. A smoker has the same problem with cigarettes, an alcoholic the same problem with a bottle. Those habits, those behaviors, those attitudes become second nature to us, and they are very hard to recognize, confront, and defeat—if we even see them as problems at all.

Another attitude I carried around with me was an aversion to athletics. I *hated* gym! I went to the best high school in the state, with the finest athletes and superbly equipped gyms. What a change from a little church grade school with nothing close to such a program! I spent four awkward, miserable years in gym—all required—and all graded and averaged into my overall scholastic performance. I bombed gym nearly every semester. I was the one who always got to be the blocker in football; I was the one stuck out in right field where I could do no harm whenever we played baseball or softball. I was always the last one rolling down the track, the one bouncing *off* the trampoline. In short, gym was not fun. I stayed clear of the ''jocks'' and avoided sports whenever I could. A good meal was my preference.

I completed my college education in the field of
history at the University of Chicago, whose presi-
dent in the 1930s, Robert Hutchins, is rumored to
have said, "Whenever I get the urge to exercise, I
lie down until it goes away." I enjoyed a school
which appreciated my intellectual athletics, while not
forcing me to participate in the humiliation of sports.

Gradually, however, I began to have a dim awareness that I was in terrible shape and looked worse. I
consistently weighed in at 215 pounds in college—
except after my first year at U. of C., when I actually sank below 200 pounds. I studied more than I
ate that year, but I must have studied well and eaten
poorly. I had the highest grade point average I ever
got there. But I looked so pale and wan at the end of
the year that, arriving at my parents' house for
summer break, my mother shrieked, "You look terrible!" and promptly set a plate of chocolate chip
cookies and a pitcher of milk before me. So much
for diet.

I tried running during one summer of my college
years, and did well. But a return to study put my
running career to a quick and breathless end.

In college I also began to develop my skills as a
gourmet cook, even teaching a class in cooking at a
local supermarket. A great hobby, but consuming
the leftovers just intensified my problem.

Seminary was no better for my body. For those
years I journeyed to the South and quickly developed
an affinity for fried chicken and pecan pie, a lethal
caloric combination. Add to that a sedentary life of
study at a small-town pace, and you have a recipe
for dietetic disaster. Cafeteria food never has lent

itself to sensible eating, as any student knows. This dining hall was no exception. By the end of my three-year seminary training, I topped out at my upper limit of 225 pounds.

The fellow across the hall from me in the dorm shared my predicament; we became known as the "wide buddies" ("one a 747, the other a DC-10"). Seminary can be an intense time of study which, for an eater, makes an intense time for munching, too. One would think that, in the life of a school of theology, the faculty members and staff would stress proper care for oneself before going into full-time ordained ministry. But how many ministers do you know who could stand to lose more than just a few pounds? I wasn't alone. I've worked subsequently with theological students in my church's geographical area, and I have noticed a heaviness, not only of soul, but especially of body, in a number of them.

Preparing to leave seminary at the end of the third year brought on the munching urge in me more than ever—especially those last few weeks of school. As I was saying good-bye to one family with whom I had become particularly close, the husband, Jim, a seminary classmate of mine, gave me a big hug. Here was a fellow in his early forties in good shape, content and able to play sports with ease, who had begun to encourage me to do something about this body God had given me. Just before we all left, Jim pulled me aside and looked me straight in the eye. Normally a man of good humor, he was as serious as I had ever seen him. "Karen and I love you too much. Lose some weight. We don't want you dead of a heart attack at forty."

I tried to pass off his remark as coming from a rabid sports enthusiast, but I could not forget his words. They echoed within me—and there was a lot of me within which to echo! "You're going to die at forty. Don't die at forty! Don't *let* yourself die at forty!"

Before long I traveled to the Chicago area to accept my first call as an assistant pastor. I was nearly out of breath from the difficult move (down four flights, up three, 700 miles in between, three round trips) and nearly out of clothes from being heavier than ever. I knew, deep within, that I had come to the point of confrontation with this demon of weight-gain. I had to do something! But I hardly knew where to begin.

I could run; I had run before and it had done some good, but I was really too heavy now to begin safely. I could diet, but I had read in *The Runner's Handbook,* by Bob Glover and Jack Shepard, that diets by themselves were not enough. Dieting only turns a fat, weak person into a thin, weak person. No real change is effected in the body, no curbing of lifelong, inbred habits. Where could I begin? I struggled in prayer for some direction from God.

God had healed me from within in so many ways already. With his help, I had worked through many personal and spiritual problems during the time I was in seminary. During my undergraduate days, I had struggled with and learned to live with my singleness. I had begun to understand that God really did love me; and then, as I experienced an unmistakable sense of calling to the ministry, my faith grew further. I had encountered Jesus Christ personally, and through his day-by-day guidance, I gained self-confidence and an ever-increasing call to serve God and his people. I *liked* myself for the first time, and tasted the glorious joy of God's inner peace. But what was my body saying to the world?

Bodies convey a lot of information about an individual and his or her self-concept—and God-concept. At that point, my interior redecoration hardly matched my exterior decor. I knew that if God had accomplished such tremendous inner healing and strengthening, he could also accomplish that outwardly. So I began to pray, not just for the success of some crash diet or exercise binge, but for a real conversion of my point of view on exercise and food. I prayed for God's Spirit to reshape not just my body, but my attitudes *about* my body, and to give me some discernment about a total program to change my outer life.

Within a couple of days, I happened to see a health club ad with a particular emphasis on "total fitness." It also advertised "No Dues Till the End of Summer"! So, no doubt with mixed motivations, I discovered myself opening the door to an entirely new experience. I felt afraid and excited, as though I were on the threshold of a new me.

On my initial trip to the club, I entered the lobby and found myself gazing around at the bright, pleasant interior. There was an ever-present strain of soft rock music in the background. This was unlike any gym I remembered! I walked up to the young woman and man at the desk. They were both young, fresh, and fit looking. I self-consciously blurted out,

"Do you still have that special deal?"

"Sure do," the man answered, "for just one more day." He looked at me for a moment and said, "Where are you a pastor?"

I wondered for a minute how he knew I was a minister—when I suddenly remembered I was wearing my clerical collar. It was probably one of the few they had seen in the place since it opened. I sure must have been nervous to forget how I was dressed!

"My name is Joe." He smiled. "I'm a Christian," he said softly.

This was more than I had prayed for. "Thank you, Lord," I breathed. Somehow, I knew that Joe would understand. I took his outstretched hand. "I want to get rid of this weight. Can you help me?"

"You can do it with God's help," he said, "—and your own hard work. We provide the equipment and teach you how to use it. Then it's up to you."

I love a challenge, and if ever there were one ahead of me, this was it!

"I want to try," I said. I was already beginning to feel better about it all. Joe gave me a tour of the club, and I was encouraged to see other economy-size men and women working away on the machines.

I must admit feeling intimidated by all of the equipment, as I had never taken the time to learn what exercise machines were supposed to do *for* me. I only knew what equipment usually did *to* me. Every time a drill instructor (disguised as a gym teacher) made me work out on such equipment, I felt hurt, tired, and generally unpleasant. However, this time I was determined to learn these machines, to understand their purposes, their uses, their benefits. For the first time, I was intrigued.

"I want you to take a test," Joe said, pointing to a portable metal step. "It's a stress test. Just walk up and down twice every five seconds, for three minutes, and then we'll take your heart rate and recovery rate—how fast your heart returns to its normal rate."

"What is my normal rate?" I asked with some apprehension. I knew it would be bad.

He frowned as he took my resting pulse. "It's pretty high. You're in extremely poor shape, according to our chart."

The verdict had been read. I felt like the defendant who had put up a great defense of excuses, knowing all along that he was guilty as charged—or as *weighed,* in this case. I submitted to the truth.

"OK, start the step test!" So I began a rhythmic bounce up and down. *I might as well be climbing my three flights of stairs at home,* I thought. I began to grunt and sweat a little more, and after only a minute and a half, I was breathing hard. I had already climbed my steps at home, and then some. Now it was the Empire State Building! I had never worked so hard on such a simple athletic task for three consecutive minutes. Afterward, I flopped down onto the step, exhausted, and Joe read off the heart rate for each ten seconds over a minute's time. He sounded like a judge reading off successive life sentences to a convicted criminal. "Twenty-six, twenty-four, twenty-four, twenty-two." At the end of a minute, it was down to a whopping 112 beats per minute, after just a three-minute step test—and I still hadn't reached my normal rate. Could I ever really work that rate down to a good, healthy level?

"OK, now we're going to measure you, and take your fat percentage," Joe said. I felt like telling him that he needn't bother—that I already knew I was 100 percent fat.

The measurements actually embarassed me further. I was a whopping 42 " in the waist, 13 " in the upper arm, 27 " in the thighs, 44 " in the obliques, the hip and "spare tire" section of the body. Using these awful measurements, as well as my weight (225 pounds), and some constants and standard body fat percentages, he began to calculate my body's fat makeup, a crucial figure I needed to know in order to bring the percentage down to a healthy level. I was a little mystified by the calculation process. (I had the same attitude toward math as I did to athletics. That changed too—but that's another story.)

"Your fat percentage is 29 percent, John," he said flatly. "That's pretty bad."

I knew that. I thought about nearly one third of my body being pure *fat,* like gelatin. God had given me this body to care for and work with. But wasn't there some operation a doctor could do that would be easier on me than all this exercise?

"I've seen some other guys do what you'll need to do," he said cautiously. "But you have a lot of work ahead of you." He must have sensed my weariness in facing the effort that lay ahead of me.

"Come on! I'll show you the machines, how to

use them, and what they will do for your body."
Finally, someone would reveal to me the mysteries
of this exercise equipment.

I went into the locker room and changed into gym
clothes for the first time in years. I remembered how
much I detested places like this in high school. I
even remembered my very first gym class in fourth
grade. I was the last one into the gym because I
couldn't tie my shoelaces—I was so awkward. And
then I was the first one "out" in sockball, a game in
which one team aims a large rubber ball at the other
team members; if you're hit, you're out. As these
scenes crossed my mind, I prayed, "Lord, redeem
these painful memories and heal me. Just get me
going and, most of all, send your Spirit to encourage
me." And slowly his peace began to fill me. I was
dressed and ready to return to the exercise area. I
was about to become an athlete—of sorts.

There were ten different machines which formed
what the club called a "circuit," and the idea is that
one goes through the circuit three times a day, three
times a week, after riding a stationary bike for fifteen minutes to get the old heart ticking safely at a
higher rate. Several of the machines were weighted;
they're called "progressive resistance machines"—
the stronger one becomes, the more weight is set to
be lifted, and the more resistance it provides. Thus
your muscles grow stronger.

As I had never used this equipment before, I
started with very light weights. The key was the
number of repetitions in a thirty-second period
(usually twelve to fifteen). That's what would help

the heart rate come way down over time, since one would work intensively for a short period and then rest for fifteen seconds. I learned that this kind of exercise is also a very efficient method of burning calories and using carbohydrates—which is the key to weight loss.

The first machine I met was the leg press, on which I was seated with my legs extended forward as I pushed upward a certain amount of weight. I could tell what level was safe for me—green markers indicated the beginners' level (blue was for intermediates and red for *real men)*. Joe demonstrated for me the proper method of the machine's use, and I tried it. I felt like a real weakling. I definitely was green! I found an amount of weight compatible with my ability, and repeated the motion ten times.

Such was the case with nearly every other machine—the arm curls, in which you're seated and pull a bar to the chin as you curl your arms toward you (the bar is connected to a certain amount of weight); the full arm press, in which you're seated on a stool and push the weight up until the arms are fully extended (that one is a killer!); the pull-up bench, in which you're face down on a half bench, ankles hooked in back, hips supported by the bench and stomach, chest and head extended out and down, alternately, and you use your back muscles to help pull you up to look at the ceiling (or stars in your eyes!), keeping stomach muscles tight.

These were followed by the military bench press, which sounds as intimidating as it really is at first. You're on your back, and, using your arms, you press toward the ceiling two bars (one for each

hand) connected to weights. This motion firms up
your chest and arms.

From there, I moved to the "deltoid," which,
rather than being a space-age robot, is a machine
that works the deltoid area in your back. Seated on a
chair, you place the back of your upper arms on two
pads and push back the weight until the pads meet.

Then I went to the overhead chair, in which,
seated, you place your elbows as well as the palms
of your hands on pads; your arms are bent at a 45°
angle. You push up on the pads, lifting over your
head a bar which is connected to weights, until your
arms are fully extended. It does wonders for your
shoulders and stomach!

From there, I went to the leg curl machine. I lay
on my stomach on a bench and hooked my ankles on
two pads connected to a pulley, which was connected to the weight. You curl your legs until you
can about reach your behind. This movement benefits leg muscles. Clearly, this point was a weak link
for me; I barely lifted the minimum weight fifteen
times. From there I went to the Roman Chair, a
chair with no seat (I never said that this was
logical!). Crossing your feet at your ankles, arms
supported by pads, you lift your knees to your chest.
Fifteen times. Impossible!

I was getting pretty woozy by now, but I hung in
there for the last stop—the sit-up bench. Joe showed
me the proper way to do a sit-up, though I tried to
tell him I didn't think I had ever learned the *im-
proper* way. So I lay down on the bench and nearly
conked out! But Joe was there to give me a little
push. *One! Two!* I struggled for the third and barely

lifted my body. *Three!* I tried for number four, but I had nothing left in me to give. "I've got to stop!" I cried out to Joe.

"OK, get back on the bike and cool down," he said as he helped me up. Before I started over there, he took my heart rate.

"It's 190 beats," he said as he wrote it down on the record card he had begun to keep for me. "Two hundred is the limit for safety. You've got to get that rate down, and you *will* if you follow this routine."

"You mean today?" I gasped as I began to push the pedals on the bike. I wondered if I could even walk back to the car, I felt so awful.

"No, you've had it for now. Just be consistent and you'll see and feel the improvement pretty soon. Don't get discouraged! It'll take time." His smile by itself was encouraging to me. "I'll meet you downstairs in a few minutes and we'll set some goals for you."

"OK," I wheezed. But I could feel the rate coming down, and, in a few minutes, I felt better. Afterward I showered up and returned to Joe's office.

When I got there, he laid out the entire program for me—more supervision in the use of the equipment; goals to lose weight and girth and to reach a lower heart rate over one, two, and three months; and the contract, payment schedule, and temporary health club card. I would aim to reach 200 pounds in three months. I would set, as my goal, to get my heart rate down so as to be in satisfactory condition. These looked like impossible goals to reach, but I remembered that God loves impossibilities. With his help, I could do these things and achieve my goals. I would also need the support of people like Joe.

While I was in his office, he said, "Why don't we pray." I sensed the Spirit's presence as we committed my regimen as well as the ultimate result to the Lord. In Joe I could observe a man who had been a proper steward of the body God had given him. I prayed for Joe and his ministry of encouragement, thankful for his personal concern about my condition. And I prayed about the tremendous opportunity God was giving me to enter such a "secular" setting as the health club. I wanted to be a witness for him in my time spent there.

Strengthened by Joe's prayers and concern, I took the goals he had set for me, as well as my contract (rather costly, which would discourage me from quitting) and my membership card and set out for the parking lot. I knew that, somehow, God had reached out and touched me and, in a new and wonderful way, was changing me forever.

So I set about incorporating visits to the health club into my weekly pastoral schedule. I made these exercise sessions a regular appointment on my calendar so that they could not get squeezed out by anything other than emergencies. Gone were the big lunches to which I had (literally) *grown* accustomed. In their place was a new discipline, dedicated to God's glory, which I had undertaken.

A workout was to become one of the most important appointments I would keep. Aside from the occasional emergency, I never missed one. The standard discipline of a three-times-a-week period of exercise was developed by this club over many years, based on the experiences of many people. If I wanted to realize the results and get the benefits promised by the club's literature, I needed to follow its direction. I became convinced that I was being a very wise steward of my time in making these visits. They were not a luxury or a leisurely pursuit for me.

Getting into shape was essential to my effectiveness as an ordained minister. I needed to take care of myself, to reorder my priorities. I could never truly care for others and their needs if I were unaware of my own needs. My friend Jim's parting words to me returned: *"We don't want you to die at forty!"* What kind of ministry could I have if I were dead?

The health club soon became part of my work routine. Those first four weeks were painful, exhausting, and what was worse—seemingly fruitless. It took every ounce of reserve, will, and prayer to keep me going when I began to feel tired or faint, sometimes even nauseated—and when the scale did not reveal much of anything in weight loss. I began to understand, however, that it had taken me twenty-five years to get out of shape. I could never expect to get into shape and to develop my body properly after only a month's time. I did achieve at least one goal during that time: I was coming to the club consistently and, for a few fleeting moments, was actually enjoying the challenge, particularly as I began to lift the weights a little more easily with each visit.

The first month's remeasurements revealed a little bit of progress. I had lost three pounds; my waist had trimmed by a couple of inches, and my heart rate had really begun to improve. I had made it to the "poor" level of fitness. I refused to be discouraged, remembering the words of some old blues song: "Been feelin' so bad that anything else feels better!"

TWO
A BRAND
NEW LIFE

The summer I discovered the health club plan and began to work out, I had been ordained a deacon in the Episcopal Church. At that time I set some goals for the date when I would be ordained a priest in the church, which was December of that year. I had about five months to reach some good goals, and a focal event toward which to devote my exercise efforts. To have a clear aim or event in mind helped me to work all the harder and more consistently.

I mentioned my goals to some people in the parish, and several of them encouraged me and entered into prayer with me as I began. I believed that I could lose all of the weight I needed to lose before the ordination—the most important event of my entire life, the confirmation of my specific calling to serve God and his church.

I began to need less and less supervision from the health club workers as I learned to keep track of my records, to estimate how much weight and repetition I needed on each machine, and to check my own heart rate to be sure I wasn't overdoing. I got to know the workers, and they would offer me specific encouragement and some tips on using the machines more effectively. I learned that many people dropped out of the program in the first four weeks, and that I already had passed a crucial point in the process. I could achieve!

One of these instructors who gave special encouragement and shared his enthusiasm with me was Dave Mills. "Crazy Dave" had an infectious optimism and just the right kind of drive to help me along as I struggled to meet my goals. He became a friend to me and picked up on my strong points as I exercised—he was the first athletic person I had ever known to do that. Maybe "jocks" could be decent people after all!

Dave came along at that crucial time toward the end of the first six months, when the results of the discipline I had taken on were just beginning to show. He knew when to push me to try a little harder to build strength. He also knew how to make exercise fun. He was always getting me through the circuits, timing all of us at the top of his voice for each thirty seconds. One day I was huffing and puffing away, but with more weight to lift on the machines than I had ever attempted. As I struggled to lift more and more on the military bench press, he stood over me and said, "Exercise—who needs it?" I could have bopped him in the nose right then!

Slowly the weight began to drop off my body—about ten pounds altogether, during the five-month period just before my ordination. I hadn't lost very *much* weight and had come nowhere near the goals I had set with Joe. But I knew that I *felt* better than I had in a long time, and I was actually getting through the day without the intense desire to take a nap or to rest. I definitely had more energy and strength.

I began to see that I would need to take on another tactic in order to lose weight. You see, as a person begins to exercise, the decreasing weight of fat is offset by the increasing weight of muscle. I wanted to look slim and trim. The image of the muscleman just didn't fit me; and, I thought, a pastor who looks like a gargantuan wrestler might threaten some of the more timid members of the congregation. Also, I just couldn't see staying around 210 pounds for the rest of my life.

The Christmas holidays loomed, however, and I knew that, were I even to consider looking at a diet, I would need to wait until these times of temptation and inevitable weight gain had passed. Diets never had appealed to me, and I carried an innate distrust of diet fads. The writers of such books always seemed to make outrageous claims for the results of their particular regimen. And a lot of diets seemed unnatural to me—like eating three pounds of pineapple, or sticking to wheat germ for two weeks, or drinking liquid formulas. To counteract my suspicion, I saw that I had to do some research on diets in order to find one I could manage while continuing to exercise. Again, a diet by itself changes a fat, weak body into a thin, weak body. I wanted to become both thin *and* strong.

Most of all, I needed to pray about this new discipline of diet. I didn't want to lose weight merely for the sake of weight loss. I wanted to make the most out of the body which God had given me. Old attitudes about eating now needed to come under the scrutiny of God's holiness. I wanted to take on this new regimen in order to glorify God and be a better steward. Dieting would be as much a spiritual as a physical discipline. Thus, I attempted to surround dieting with a cloak of prayer and faith that God would encourage a spirit of self-control within me. He has promised that as a spiritual gift.

I continued to exercise throughout the holidays and, to my astonishment, I didn't gain a pound, but even lost a couple more! During the month of January, I went on a retreat for a week and devoted time to preparing to diet, change old habits, and adopt a new way of life. I continued to read while on retreat, praying over each diet, looking at the benefits and the drawbacks to each one, and examining how each treated eating habits. I began to say farewell to certain kinds of foods as God worked some final healing of my spirit in preparation for taking on the rigors of dieting.

There is a period of time observed in some Christian churches which is called Lent. It consists of forty days leading up to Easter, during which Christians are called upon to ponder Christ's death and work on the cross, with particular attention to spiritual disciplines. Often it involves taking on some good work as a result of faith, giving up something in self-denial, or altering some behavior that needs changing. The forty days are based on Jesus' fasting and prayer in the wilderness for forty days before beginning his ministry in Galilee. They offer an opportunity to participate in his life and work through personal sacrifice. I began to sense that Lent would be an ideal time to take on the combined disciplines of diet and exercise. I believed God's Spirit would enable me to stick to my plan during that period of time, and I eagerly anticipated some spiritual growth besides. I was getting excited about going on a diet—and this from a person who was a professional food enthusiast!

I settled on the Scarsdale Diet of Dr. Herman Tarnower as the program which would benefit me the most. (I'll say more in chapter seven about choosing a diet.) In Tarnower's diet, starches, fried foods, and breads are eliminated and a rigorous and very simple menu is substituted for a two-week period. Then a maintenance diet is prescribed for two weeks, after which time one may return to the diet until his or her final goal is achieved. On the diet, made up of a good balance of fruits, vegetables, and meat, one never has more than 1,500 calories a day, yet the amount of food is ample and quite normal and sensible.

Every body is different and reacts differently to diets, so I was careful not to take the weight-loss claims too seriously. I merely set a goal for myself of 180 pounds, a weight I had not seen in ages. As I prepared to go on this diet, I bought food very carefully to include only what was needed for the two weeks, and I cleared out of my house every last bit of nondiet food, so as to avoid temptation. I bought a scale to measure my weight daily. Going on a diet takes spiritual, physical, and psychological preparation.

I set the target date on which I would begin my

new way of eating and my new thinking about food.
In churches that observe Lent, Ash Wednesday
marks the beginning of the forty-day period of
denial, devotion, and discipline to the Lord. It's
called Ash Wednesday because on that day Christians focus upon their mortality and the basic sinful
nature of humankind in light of the great holiness of
our God and his call to us to live sober and holy
lives. We say, "Dust you are, and to dust you shall
return."

What better way to begin this discipline than to
commit it to God's care, to submit to him saying, "I
can't seem to control my eating, Lord. I want to be
a good steward both of food and of the body you
have given me. I can't do it on my own, but with
your help, I *can* learn to be disciplined."

People sometimes think that pastors have great
self-control. I opened myself to my congregation,
saying quietly among a few of my trusted members
that I was beginning this effort and that I wanted
them to be praying with me in my struggle. With
their support, a recognition of my sinfulness, lack of
discipline, and poor self-image before God, and with
the hope of improving, I began to pray and to eat
with care.

Actually, except for the absence of desserts and
starches, the diet was not a jarring departure
from normal eating. It was plain and simple and
marked out exactly—no discretion allowed for the
weak-willed! But I could eat abundantly what was on
the plan. There were days when a very low-
carbohydrate, low-calorie plan for eating, combined

with vigorous exercise, left me feeling worn out—particularly toward the end of the period. But generally I felt better and better and had more than enough energy to make it through a busy pastor's day.

I made it a point not to schedule lunches out for business—I'd meet people for coffee instead. When any dinner engagement was planned, I made it clear that I *needed* to be on this diet and that I would be happy to bring my own food. I wanted no one to make a fuss over me, but this condition was one I imposed when I was a guest in a home. I went to no restaurants during that time, which did wonders for my budget. People saw quite a lot of me, since I did not cut myself off from social contact. I went on with life as usual, except that I packed lunches and dinners to take wherever I went. Most people hardly gave it a second thought—or they were intrigued, and then supportive of my efforts.

The first two weeks passed. I lost ten pounds! I was actually down to 200, and I began to see a decline *daily* when I would weigh in! I praised God that finally I could begin to see some results. I now went on the maintenance diet for two weeks, which was a little more elaborate and included a few things not permitted on the strict diet. I lost *ten more pounds* and I was feeling great!

Twenty pounds in four weeks, down to a little under 190! I began to notice that my clothes were a little baggy here and there, and that I was beginning to fit (very snugly) into a few things which I hadn't worn for some time. I was within ten pounds of my goal, and I knew that I could make it. God had blessed me so richly and had strengthened my own will.

A few people began to notice the change that was coming over me, although many could not discern exactly what was happening to me. "You look thinner, John—are you feeling all right?" was the most common expression of interest and concern. I began to babble on about how well this diet was working for me, with the help of exercise. Soon word began to spread through the congregation that the associate pastor was losing weight. Some more people became enthusiastic, and several more began to pray with me. They shared their own personal struggles with overeating and I was humbled by their honesty. *I'm not the only one who has faced this temptation,* I thought.

I returned to the stricter diet for another two weeks. At first, nothing seemed to happen. I stayed at 187 for several days, and I began to wonder whether something was wrong. As I teetered on the edge of initial discouragement, the weight began to peel off daily once again: 185, 183, 182, 181, 180! And 179 and 177 and—wait a minute!

I surpassed my goal. My body wasn't prepared to quit after those two weeks. I had a hunger *to lose more weight,* not to eat. Now, mind you, I had not the slightest fear of obsession about losing weight. My body simply had not reached the point where it wanted to stop, and one look in the mirror revealed that, for my particular physical frame, I could afford to lose some more weight. I had begun to fit comfortably into clothes I never thought I could wear, and the clothes which I had been wearing I could wear no longer.

For a church group meeting one evening, I slipped into a pair of jeans and a tapered shirt which I first literally had to dust off (the clothes had not seen the light of day for so long). "You are getting *so thin,*" one of the members said. "You're really an inspiration to me!" Jan knew just how difficult weight loss could be, and her encouragement did more to lift my spirits that night than any comment anyone had yet made.

Easter came that year, a grand celebration with a careful meal I prepared for my family, who had not seen me since I began weight loss. They were shocked at first. I had wondered whether my mother would gasp and make some comment about my health and well-being. Instead, she hugged me and said, "You look better than ever!"

I began to tell them all excitedly about my experience in dieting, and how wonderful I felt to surrender this part of my life to the Lord's healing touch. My parents and brothers and sister all stood with me in my efforts and encouraged me to continue. And so, even though both the target date and weight loss had been surpassed, I decided to shoot for 170 pounds as a safe and realistic weight for someone nearly six feet tall. I continued to feel fine and have increasing amounts of energy, so I had no reservations about continuing.

You may be asking by now—particularly if you are a health professional—whether or not I was under a doctor's supervision during this period of exercise and weight loss. Now, your physician might be different from mine, but the doctor whom I had seen for years told me every time I came in for a checkup, "John, lose weight." I always asked him, "How?" He would always reply, "Stop eating." I would reply, "That's all?"

That's all as far as he was concerned. That little conversation was almost like a ritual, and I no longer had patience for that indefinite kind of advice. He advised me to stop eating or to eat less, but he never was able to recommend a diet or tell me how to eat right. He never took the time to educate me about food, eating habits, and exercise, though I would ask him for specific direction.

I hope your experience is different. If it's the same, and you are nearing age thirty-five or older, or if you haven't had a regular physical checkup in several years, then it is essential that you find a physician who understands about exercise and nutrition. Ask your doctor for a specific referral to such a physician, check with your local YMCA, or with the American Running and Fitness Association, which lists sports physicians and therapists who can help you.

I had seen a physician just before graduating from seminary and returning to Chicago, and he gave me an overall clean bill of health. Several nurses in my congregation also made it part of their ministry to monitor me and to continue to check with me about how I was feeling. You might have these kinds of resources in your own church or community. All you need to do is ask. But let me reinforce the advice that, if you are older than thirty-five, or if you have not been thoroughly examined recently by a health professional, you *must* be tested before dieting so that you do not overwhelm your system. You also must educate yourself to know what exercise and nutrition are designed to accomplish, so that you can ask intelligent questions of your physician and monitor your own progress. That's what I did.

I was really in for a shock, however, when I looked in the mirror. Just a year earlier, I had been imprisoned in the world of the extra large and the ill-fitting. Now I shook my head in disbelief. I knew that I could no longer wear anything I had in my closet. I had to begin from scratch. My old clothes were useless to me now. I cleared out the closet, removing every last piece of "fat" clothing, sending some to my church's resale shop, some to the Salvation Army, and some to the trash. I could never return to those clothes.

Another essential person in my life became the tailor. You will need to get a good tailor or seamstress and watch for sales, because, if your experience is anything like mine, you'll have to buy an entirely new set of clothes. Make sure that you have a little money in the bank to do that. I was astounded when I walked into a quality clothing store near my home. I had never thought I could wear the styles I was beginning to wear.

I went to buy a new suit just as I had started to descend below 180 pounds, and found my waist had shrunk from a forty-two-inch girth to just a shade under thirty-six inches! Everything had shrunk. I had gone down two sizes in a suit coat, an inch in the neck for shirts, and, amazingly, I now comfortably wore a medium size in sport shirts. The investment I made in new clothing (a substantial one) would be yet another reason to keep off the weight. I couldn't *afford* to get fat ever again!

In late March and early April, I decided that it was safe once again to run. I had lost enough weight that my heart would not be overtaxed. My heart rate showed that I had achieved nearly a "good condition" according to the health club chart.

I enjoy running. Some find exercise to be tedious and tiring. For me, however, to leave the office in order to enjoy the quiet and the fresh air, and to experience a time when the body is working with little effort and maximum efficiency, is glorious. In fact, I think I taste heaven from time to time, as running relaxes me and opens my heart and mind to God. Some of my most fruitful times of prayer have been while running.

I began with a run of two miles, and slowly worked up to three, then gradually to more than four. I would add a block here and a block there from week to week. I found that the circuit equipment training and the running complemented each other. I would work out at the health club Monday, Wednesday, and Friday, and run Tuesday, Thursday, and Saturday, and relax after worship on Sunday.

I had begun to take up racquetball and tennis as well, so I would sometimes indulge in these sports on a quiet Sunday afternoon for a great time of fellowship with friends from church, or with other health-minded pastors in the community. In fact, one Sunday I involved my entire congregation in easy warm-up exercises as part of a sermon illustration on

Christians shaping up their bodies as well as their faith (based on 1 Corinthians 9:24-27, the text for that Sunday). I think I had the most alert congregation in the community that morning!

Within two weeks of Easter, I reached 170 pounds, and ended the diet in prayer and participation in that sacred meal, the Lord's Supper. What a spiritual strengthening I had received from this experience! I could think of no more appropriate way to begin a new life of health and fitness than to eat and drink in celebration around the Lord's Table, to partake of the Bread of Life. Now I would leave the specific discipline of diet and continue exercising. But I had learned some new principles from dieting, principles which have helped me to maintain my weight with little trouble or anxiety. I had learned an entirely new way of eating, and how to enjoy new food. I had also learned a completely new way of preparing food—cooking more simply and planning menus more carefully.

Is it as amazing to you as it is to me that, even on such a strict diet, I could still eat far better than over three-quarters of this world's population? I had far more quantity and quality of food, and a much wider selection of items from which to choose, than many human beings could ever imagine having. Sure, I felt some hunger during the diet, especially in the early stages. But it was nothing compared to the hunger which many of the world's people, particularly children, live with from day to day. Although I had worked on a diet primarily to improve my own condition, I also became aware of hunger in the world, and the wanton misuse of food by many in

Western culture, particularly Americans.

During the time I dieted and exercised, I watched as our country attempted to use food as a weapon against other nations in foreign policy wrangling. Making a weapon out of food—the very stuff of life! God's Spirit convicted me of this deep-seated sinfulness in which I had been participating and continue to participate. My social awareness increased through this experience, and I prayed that God might give me the wisdom to be a better steward of food and to be thankful for all that I do have.

For another month or so—until mid-May—I continued to lose a little bit as my body sought to find its new weight level and metabolism. In my exercise, with Joe's help, I began to work on some new machines and leave others behind in order to tone up specific areas of my body which had been neglected for so long—for example, my stomach muscles. This work was for the longer term. Muscles are strengthened gradually, with concentrated work. Toning and shaping one's body is a subtle process. Three years later, I find myself still working on it. I realize it's a lifetime discipline, a continuing effort.

While keeping an eye on the food I ate once I returned to "normal" eating patterns, and continuing to exercise, my weight came to rest at 165 pounds. For three years, that is the level at which it has been stable, sometimes shifting five or so pounds in either direction. I have learned to weigh in every day. It's like watching the gas gauge on your car—is it too full or too empty? Does the car need a tune-up? It's important.

Setting goals that one can achieve makes all the

difference. With the goal ahead, and the possibility of achievement and success, discipline comes, both physically and spiritually. So I set a goal for exercise, specifically in my running program. The town I lived in at the time had a 10-kilometer race (6.2 miles) on the Fourth of July. I decided to train for this race, the first athletic competition which I had ever dared to enter. Perhaps I could be an athlete after all!

"Do you not know that, in a footrace, every runner competes for the prize?" asks Paul in 1 Corinthians. The prize is the crown of life, the upward call of God in Christ Jesus. I believe that this crown, this goal, this *call* is what every person is meant to achieve in the life God has given him or her. As Christians we recognize, accept, endorse, and have conviction of the truth of God's call to us in Christ. We each have the ability to achieve the crown, the laurel wreath that every runner in the ancient world was allowed to wear if he won the race. God has made us all winners, and all competitors—not against one another, but against our weaknesses. God promises us success in gaining control of those habits which seem out of control, beyond our abilities to break. We can submit them to God's will in us.

Christians for too long have adopted without thinking the ancient Greek separation of body and spirit. This position declares that the spirit is all that counts: the body is merely transitory and not to be fussed over. The New Testament writers, Paul in particular, are still misunderstood over this question, and a little later on I'll look at the biblical understanding of the human body which allows the Christian to be concerned about physical *and* spiritual health at the same time.

But let it be clear that my understanding of the Christian faith and life—and of my own calling to serve in Christ's church—is that we always minister to the *whole* person. That is why I'm writing about how I have experienced his healing grace while my body—his creation—underwent a complete transformation. I am not only a different body as a result of losing sixty-five pounds. I am a different person, a different Christian for the experience.

THREE
DELIGHTING
IN FATNESS?

God doesn't care if we're fat and happy, does he?

He certainly *does* care. And is it really so likely for one to be fat and happy at the same time? While God does make the impossible happen from time to time in our lives, he doesn't uphold contradictions. And that old stereotype of the fat and happy person is just that—a contradiction and a well-worn myth.

A fat person, in fact, often can be miserable, especially if he realizes that his weight is primarily due to addictive overeating.* When a person is dealing with an addiction of any kind, be it alcohol or drugs or gambling or food, it is a serious situation. Besides the physical damage, the addiction usually also indicates a deep well of hurt, frustration, guilt, and anger. And it almost always masks a case of low self-esteem.

In my case, food had become a way of propping myself up when I really felt miserable and depressed

*Apart from a distinct medical cause in a minority of cases, overeating is the culprit.

inside. And since the good times I did have often
revolved around meals with others, the conviviality
and warmth of friendship around the dinner table
blended with my enjoyment of eating. So, when I
was alone, or friendless, or hurting, or bored—I
could eat. And when I did, a flood of warm
memories would waft into the cold room.

But I really was not happy with myself. In fact,
after I would eat (actually, "binge" or eat uncon-
trollably), I would end up more miserable than
before. And I didn't binge on foods I needed. You
wouldn't find me munching celery or carrot sticks or
other low-calorie snacks. I always went for the
chocolate-chip cookies, peanuts, french fries, chips,
and other fattening and unhealthy foods.

I wondered whether God could ever reach down
far enough to heal me and help me find happiness
within. I longed desperately to break the consumption habit that was consuming *me* and costing me my
inner peace.

One look at the average magazine rack reveals that
thin bodies are in. Overweight men and women
readers try to smile as they groan through the pages
that are proffered each month on "Losing Forty
Pounds in Forty Days," or the "No Pain, No Gain,
No Strain Fitness Program" with ninety-eight easy
exercises guaranteed to tone your entire body. I
never imagined that I could possibly look like any of
those handsome men who slithered through the pages
of fitness and happiness.

I kept looking for the "Miracle No-Work Diet."
Or maybe some method which would incorporate
limitless quantities of soft-batch double chocolate

cookies. It was treats like that which brought the most pleasure to my life. But you never see thin and fit people wolfing down plates full of cookies. Instead they smile as they eat little tins of yogurt on TV. You hardly ever see overweight people looking happy in mass-market advertising. They're the ones you see wilting without an air-conditioner, or struggling with too-small pantyhose, looking ridiculous. Fatness is not a positive image in our culture.

Nevertheless, the myth persists of the fat and happy person. I think that the most powerful image of someone fat and jolly is Santa Claus. Remember those lines in "The Night Before Christmas" about Santa shaking and laughing like a bowl full of jelly? Do you know anyone who laughs, jiggling like jelly? Perhaps someone in your own mirror. Well, what's so funny about that? Is obesity a laughing matter? Not to those who cannot seem to control their weight.

I know from my own experience that, behind the layer of laughter, there is usually a person who is deeply unhappy with himself or herself. There are some people who suffer from a medical problem—a runaway thyroid gland, or a metabolic imbalance—who cannot lose weight and seem to be consigned permanently to some level of obesity. That is very sad, and these people suffer the stigma of their looks, often experiencing mental and emotional as well as physical pain with their condition. But for the majority of people, the problem of obesity and lack of fitness is an inner condition of low self-esteem and negative self-worth.

I remember a woman who was better than one

hundred pounds overweight, whom I came to know in a group of prospective church workers. We all had to work closely together, and we became acquainted with one another's hopes and fears on a deep level. On the surface, and somewhat deeper, too, this woman always had a smile and a great sense of humor. Her laughter was infectious. I thought to myself, "How can anyone who looks like that be apparently happy?" It seemed to me that, while bringing her love and laughter to those she served, she was seriously neglecting herself.

I also noticed that she talked and talked—endlessly. She had a tremendous facility with words. When someone would ask her impressions of a case she was on, she would explain on and on in great detail. But I wondered whether she really was letting us know *her*—the person inside. Her profusion of words served as a barrier which kept the rest of us from getting through to her. She didn't seem to hear us, and we wondered if she was relating to us as her real self.

In ministering to her along with the other group members, I began to perceive an image of this woman and her condition. Her words seemed like a thick insulation surrounding her, keeping her warm and safe inside. She could hear others through the insulation, but no one could get through to her to really touch her, or to show God's love for her *to* her. Her body was the outward sign of her inner condition. Her fat was like a wall surrounding her, protecting her from the jabs and sharpness of the outside world, and keeping her from feeling the chill of possible criticism. My analysis was scary in its accuracy—because I looked at myself and saw the same condition developing.

Did I want to become completely insulated like this woman? Did I want to shut out the world?

Gradually, as we worked with this woman, the members of our group began to peel away some of her many layers of protection. We made efforts to touch her, and to demonstrate in gentle and innocent ways—such as smiles and hugs—our care for her. She seemed to welcome our persistence in loving her, until one day she broke down, weeping and pouring out how she felt—unlovable. She felt that she had nothing to offer, and could not conceive of being a beautiful person to anyone. At the core, she felt almost worthless. But she had built up a front of defense from the cold, as well as the care of others.

The sad thing was, I looked at my own life and saw the same basic problem. I knew that I would have to seek out God's love and healing in a special way if I were to deal with the root problem of my obesity—my lack of self-worth. I would have to learn how to feel, after years of protecting myself. I would have to be taught how to feel good about myself, and to receive the gifts of others, acknowledging that they were really gifts from God. And I decided that I wanted to help others find healing once I myself could lose weight.

In our culture, this level of personal stock-taking is extremely threatening to most men. Women are more accustomed, and are encouraged, to cultivate an inner life and to radiate beauty. Most men tend to be outer-directed and active, taking little time for reflection. And as a result, many men in our culture are actually emotionally handicapped. They do not know *that* they feel, much less *how* they feel. Men can think that feelings are means to the end in human relationships, rather than valuing them as part of being human—part of the divine image and plan for human life. So men do not "delight in fatness"—they are simply fat; and when they are, they usually don't give two hoots and a holler about their condition.

It is also true that men often do not perceive the impression their appearance makes on another person. They do not seem to understand that much of success and failure can depend on physical factors. Yet in many cases there are no second chances for another impression. I see overweight men send signals of unhappiness which give a destructive first impression in a sales pitch or a negotiation. The result is as if other people in the room say to themselves, "This guy looks sloppy—he's probably sloppy in his work as well." And they may be right. The man could be sloppy in his home life, his business life, and even in his spiritual life.

And yet this man—and many men are like him—is not in touch with his inner need. While men highly value physical prowess, their egos often keep them in the dark about their true physical condition. For example, a sedentary, overweight middle-aged male charges onto the softball field or the running track on any given weekend, convinced that he can do what he always did twenty years ago. When this man returns home, limping from a pulled hamstring muscle, completely worn out from the exertion, he comes to the realization that he is not the conditioned athlete he thought he was. His self-perception is totally out of proportion to his actual condition. Likewise, his perception of his feelings and what he actually believes about himself are at odds with each other.

The basic problem with many American men is that they find it difficult to admit that they have a personal problem, particularly a weight problem. Men often claim to be doing just fine—yet sport thirty extra pounds which belie their words.

Have you ever noticed that there are few books— even very few articles—written by men who have admitted to being overweight and are struggling to get in shape? Men generally are afraid to write to other men about their insecurities—and many men will not bring themselves to read a book about a depressing, "downer" subject.

So, if you are a male, I commend you for taking the important step of admitting that you have a problem with weight. You have already won a major gain in the battle for fitness. Women who read this book should understand that some women may also have difficulty admitting to problems in their lives; but women in our culture, who are encouraged to listen to their feelings and to maintain their bodies in order to be attractive, will likely have gotten at least to this point already.

In the case of the Christian man, he will realize that there is a spiritual side to life which has a bearing on this issue of fitness and wholeness. He is aware that God can heal other parts of his life—attitudes, errant desires, the lack of openness and honesty. What will follow in the remainder of this chapter is particularly related to that overall healing.

Those who are very new in their walk with the Lord, or who have not yet begun that walk, may discover they need increased strength—for the battle with being overweight is not just a matter of "losing it." It is a case of becoming a new person.

In 2 Corinthians Paul says of the Christian, and of himself, "Though we once regarded Christ [from a human point of view], we do so no longer. Therefore, if anyone is in Christ, he is a new creation; the old has gone, the new has come!" (2 Corinthians 5:16b, 17). The root of effective, permanent weight loss is far more than a plan for shedding pounds. It involves shedding an old, outdated image of oneself.

Losing weight can be a matter of tearing off the insulation around your heart, and dealing at last with that fearful, unhappy, hurt person inside. Insecurity causes many people to neglect their looks. And that neglect is evidenced in eating to excess. You cannot lose weight and become fit and whole for good until you also seek a deeper healing. In order to make the effort, you have to feel that you're worth the discipline and pain it will take to lose the weight.

There are as many ways to seek the release of your own personal burden as there are people who carry one. Some find that a group such as Overeaters Anonymous, or TOPS (Take Off Pounds Sensibly) encourages them to discover the key to their overweight condition. There are chapters of these groups just about everywhere. You need only look in the phone book to find one and join up. Some people will want to see their pastor, who may or may not understand the dynamics of obesity, par-

ticularly the spiritual implications. If a minister has
some experience in working with alcoholics, he
could be helpful, because I believe the core problem
is the same—lack of self-esteem at a deep level.
Only the physical problems or manifestations are different.

Still others may seek out a Christian therapist or
counselor who can be helpful in defining the basic
psychological problems involved. Some may engage
in self-study and reflection, or may seek to work
with a partner or close friend who can be honest and
supportive through a weight-loss and fitness program.

You may notice that I have not suggested the
family physician. I mentioned earlier the frustrating
experience that I had with my own doctor. He
always told me that I should lose weight but he
never was able to teach me how to do it. Like many
physicians, his main work was not in preventive
medicine, but in detecting and treating symptoms of
illness. It's easier for a doctor to practice that tradi-
tional method, and there is always a treatment to
prescribe for just about any symptom.

I am not suggesting that the medical profession as
a whole is negligent of preventive medicine, or is
unprepared to give nutritional advice. And I certainly suggest that you consult with your physician
before you begin a weight-loss program. But my advice is that you seek out a physician who believes in
and is adept at holistic medicine, who has an understanding of the interrelationship of physical, mental,
emotional, and spiritual factors in a physical problem
such as obesity. Few doctors have been trained in

this way, although medical schools increasingly are coming to recognize the need to treat the whole person. Medical consumers also are beginning to demand whole-person care.

A holistic physician ought to have some working knowledge of methods of physical conditioning so as to advise you how to begin your work in that area. A knowledge of nutrition would also enable the doctor to teach you sensible eating habits. You'd have a real gem of a doctor if he or she could pray with you as well!

If this all sounds like hard work and major change, you're hearing it right. It is painful and difficult to begin a program that builds in a realistic and healthy way toward permanent fitness. When I started my own program to lose weight I believed—and still do—that it is a major undertaking to examine yourself, seek healing, reach your goal, and then maintain a state of physical well-being. It takes a massive amount of prayer. Remember when the disciples attempted to cast out a demon in Jesus' name, yet met with a failure? Then Jesus healed the epileptic boy, and the disciples spoke with him privately afterward and asked, "Why couldn't we drive it out?" Jesus replied, "This kind can come out only by prayer" (Mark 9:28, 29).

Many who have struggled to lose weight and to stay in good condition can testify that they first had to acknowledge that they could never have healed themselves. God's tremendous healing power began to work in them when they asked for it, after they prayed to be healed.

Those who face the prospect of a large weight loss

for the first time, or who have tried again and again without success, need to come to the admission that they have a condition that only deep, consistent prayer—on their part and on the part of others—can resolve.

People who are overweight may become "losers," literally. They also can be winners in the end, by admitting their human frailty and facing up to their basic inability to control their own lives. They know that there are weaknesses in *every* person, and that they need God's power in a most personal way. Those who cannot admit human failing and lack of control over their lives are the real losers in the end.

People who persevere and lose weight will find that, with God, they are winners, because God made them in his image, and it is good. Although that image has become marred in every human life by some problem, people have found visible, impressive victory and release. They can testify effectively to God's divine power.

God's image in us ought to be evidenced in wholeness and fitness—physical, emotional, moral, and mental. God does give us all the potential for fitness, but striving to attain it means contending with what Dr. Scott Peck (in his book *The Road Less Traveled*) has identified as the principal problem in human life today: *spiritual laziness.* Only God can heal us of this affliction, if we would exert ourselves and dare to ask for his help.

God desires that we be our best for him, and that we be active for him. With his help we can be fit Christians, not *fat* Christians. He gives us the ability, through the Spirit, to overcome our weaknesses.

But we must begin by being honest with ourselves and with God. That means first taking stock of ourselves and our behavior. It involves repentance and renewal, which are gifts from God. Yet we cannot appreciate them in their fullness unless we take responsibility for ourselves.

So how does one go about reforming from being a heavyweight? How does one take stock and actually begin the mental, emotional, and spiritual preparation for losing weight?

Personal reflection begins, literally, in a mirror. . . .

FOUR
THE
SPRAWLING
TEMPLE

When you take that good, long look in the mirror—a floor-length mirror is most helpful—the first thing you exercise may be your eyes. They may bulge in disbelief. That's because you are taking the first honest look at the body God has given you—and what you have done with it. Your body is not meant to be like the talents in Jesus' parable; it wasn't intended to grow larger with time!

So you're large. You're not the first person who has ever been out of shape, out of condition. As you look at yourself in the mirror and contemplate what is ahead of you, you need to do a little bit of long-range planning. If you see a body that is terribly out of shape, you must understand that your transformation into a fit, conditioned, and controlled-weight person is not going to happen overnight. The best weight loss is not instant.

Wouldn't it be simpler, we think, if we were tubs of lard—then a little heat could melt us down to exactly the size we wanted to be. The body, fortunately, is not built on this principle. There are overweight people in sunny Phoenix just as there are in Philadelphia.

Just as you are getting a truthful look in the mirror, I want you to put away all pictures of athletes and those debonair models in the magazine ads. You will not look the way they do. Every human body is different. There is no *perfect* body to which you can aspire—there is only the well-conditioned body which potentially is yours. You are one of a kind and special—therefore, your way to conditioning and your need for shaping up will be different from anyone else's.

We all were created uniquely by Almighty God, with different needs and different potentials. You can live up to your potential, with God guiding you all along the way. After all, he is the Master Builder, the one who holds the blueprints. As David says, "You [God] created my inmost being; you knit me together in my mother's womb. I praise you because I am fearfully and wonderfully made; your works are wonderful, I know that full well" (Psalm 139:13, 14). Do you accept that Bible truth as applying to you?

God's blueprints are for temples, places of worship which are divinely ordained and designed. The Temple in Jerusalem was, to the Jews, the very place where God dwelt in his fullness. It is there that he was worshiped by devout Jews many times a year. So when Paul says that we are temples of the Holy Spirit, he means that we are to honor God in our physical bodies. He reminds the men and women of the Corinthian church, "Do you not know that your body is a temple of the Holy Spirit, who is

in you, whom you have received from God? You
are not your own; you were bought at a price.
Therefore honor God with your body" (1 Corinthians 6:19, 20). And Paul doesn't mean a price per
pound.

To put it another way: God said that he wants us
to be his temples, not his convention centers. I am
reminded of the old convention center in San Fran-
cisco—the Cow Palace. Think about it. What kind of
a temple are we?

I live in an older home. When I moved into it,
much of the lovely woodwork had been painted
over, the hardwood floors were an ugly yellow, the
dining room was an utter disaster, and the finished
basement was filthy from years of disuse. On the
outside, I needed to put on new shutters and take out
overgrown shrubbery. Eventually the heating plant
will have to be replaced. There's a lot of work to be
done in this house.

The problem is, there are no plans available, no
blueprints for the house. There is no other house
quite like it in all of Chicago. As I did a little
research on it, I came across some old records in
City Hall which detailed the work that the general
contractor had done when he built it. I didn't have
the house plans, but I did have some idea of how it
was put together. Gradually, I am able to figure out
how the planned renovations will fit this particular
house.

Getting into physical shape poses similar problems. We do not have our own specific "body blueprints" that we can return to in planning renovation,
but we do have certain biblical principles which sug-

gest what our Maker intended for us. We need only to be faithful to him in our efforts at renovation, and to realize that hard work is ahead of us.

Having said that each of us is unique, and that there is no perfect body, I'm going to eat—no, take back—my words a little. Actually, there are three basic body types: *mesomorphs, ectomorphs,* and *endomorphs.** These terms refer to three types of physiques: sinewy, stringy, or burly. The *mesomorph,* or the sinewy man, has well-developed musculature and minimal body fat. That's about 20 percent of the male population. Then there are the 20 percent who are *ectomorphs.* They are stringy, often tall and linear in appearance, not having strong musculature. Sometimes they are Slim Jims—but when they gain weight, it is very noticeable, because there is not a strong muscle or bone to fill out.

Yes, I've been saving the bad news. Most of us with the weight problems are in that 60 percent of the male population who are *endomorphs.* We're burly, and we have a tendency therefore to have a soft and round physique. Unless we're careful to work out, we develop prominent abdominal sag, fleshiness in our thighs, buttocks, and arms, and we carry a large amount of body fat.

You cannot change your body type—but you can work with the God-given potential of your body type. I know loads of thin, slight men who would give all that they have—which is not much, weight-wise—to gain good muscle structure and some bulk.

It's not like real estate; there's no way to trade

*My application here applies mainly to men.

your body for a different style. I have to make the most of what I have. So do you.

So go back to that mirror again and determine your body type. Now you understand why you should be looking at your reflection and not at your favorite athlete. You see, *your* best look and best conditioning will not necessarily be someone else's. So accentuate *your* individuality. Build *your* potential. Because if you try to be someone you physically cannot be, you will be forever frustrated. God did not make us to be frustrated like that. He desires for us to be fit in our own bodies.

If you have an attitude of acceptance as you begin to condition yourself, then you will succeed. You will start out flabby, perhaps, but as you exercise and diet sensibly, you will see that flab disappear. What's more, your physical shortcomings will fade away as you shape up generally. Your temple will grow more and more to resemble the Architect's original plan—for you.

This may be the first time that you really have taken a look at your physical resources. Lurking behind that flab is a terrific looking, well-conditioned body. You'll surprise yourself!

I had been working out steadily for almost a year when I happened to take an extended look at myself in the mirror. You can understand that I had always felt ashamed to look in the mirror, because I knew what a sad sight I was. I tell you, this time I did a double take! My arms were strong and muscular—veins visible from shoulder to wrist! Stomach and abdomen—naturally tight and lithe! Love handles—gone! (I really cheered for that one.) Neck—taut and firm, lacking a double-decker chin! This image in the mirror was real! It was what I was meant to look like all along. I drew in a deep breath and, exhaling, said, "Praise God—that's the person I was meant to be!"

It does get harder with age to get rid of the sag, but it is not impossible. Basically our body patterns are pretty well set by age thirty, so if you are over thirty, you'll have a somewhat more difficult road ahead of you. But don't despair. It's never too late to get into shape. Who knows—you could end up better conditioned after your program than many people are in their twenties.

Another fellow named John frequented the health club where I was a member. He was sixty-two years old and a grandfather three times. He began his program in his early fifties, after his first—and only—heart attack. Without fail, he would come in to do his sit-ups, work the machines, and stretch his short, mesomorphic body. He wasn't Mr. America—but John was in as good a shape as I've seen a man his age, given his limitations set by his doctor.

And there was Hal, who was in his early seventies, yet worked out hard three times a week. He looked—and felt—younger than anyone could imagine. He simply was a steady worker in his program.

Bill was in his early forties and would get out of shape during the winter months when his construction work would slack off. He, like me, was a classic endomorph, and his work only accentuated his burliness. Instead of a slim-and-trim look, Bill opted for a muscular look which suited his particular height and build, as well as his personality. He, too, was in good condition.

So, you see, age doesn't matter, except that there are sometimes more years of inactivity to overcome. But it can be done—men do it all the time. And they all have to start *somewhere*. Maybe at the Cow Palace, after all!

You'll have to take a long look too at your companion, the refrigerator. All of your intentions and actions to condition yourself will be for naught if you do not confront your eating habits as well.
If you have been able to isolate why you eat the way you do, then you will be able to take steps to control your eating, dieting sensibly and carefully, if necessary.

In order for a diet to work effectively, it must contain three elements:

First, it must sound sensible. Even if your eating habits are poor, you can probably see the foolishness in eating fourteen mangoes and five carrots for a day's intake. The old adage works here two ways. If it looks foolish, it probably is—and if its promises seem too good to be true, they probably are.

Second, a diet must be easy to prepare. You guarantee yourself undue frustration if you pursue a diet that requires 14.3858432 ounces of chopped celery cooked for 3.825 minutes in an oven set at 333°. Avoid the hassle.

Third, the foods specified should be those that would be in any well-balanced diet, leaving off an occasional item that is particularly caloric. You'll have enough trouble maintaining a good spirit as you diet, so why trouble yourself further with impossible dietary demands?

That's the outer form of the diet. The inner "soul" of the diet process means setting long-range goals for your weight loss, but working diligently on the short-term aspects. You must not become obsessed with dieting, nor must you throw up your hands if it doesn't seem to bring immediate results. In either case, you are not in control—your defeatist attitudes are. So keep the long-range goal in mind, but strive only for today.

Jesus' principle of anxiety reduction is important for us to claim here as we prepare to go on a diet: "Therefore I tell you, do not worry about your life, what you will eat or drink; or about your body, what you will wear. Is not life more important than food, and the body more important than clothes?" (Matthew 6:25). Jesus invites us to set new priorities for our lives, to live for him in a new way. He will help us and reassure us.

"Look at the birds of the air; they do not sow or reap or store away in barns, and yet your heavenly Father feeds them. Are you not much more valuable than they? Who of you by worrying can add a single hour to his life?" (vv. 26, 27). Or take off a single inch? Or lose a single pound?

My friend Carl weighs in at 210 pounds and is always trying one diet or another. He'll lose a few pounds quickly, but gain them back as soon as he's off the diet. Diets are an endless round of frustration for Carl precisely because he does not prepare to lose weight. He does not *prepare to be a loser,* if you will. He *is* a loser—in the battle to get weight off and get into condition. He cannot stick to a diet precisely because he has neither a long-range goal nor a short-term method.

Dieting is a whole new way of life with its own set of choices and challenges. When you start a regimen you are changing some very subtle, and very powerful, patterns of behavior. You are altering certain psychological and spiritual associations you have held concerning food and your body. These behaviors die hard. Satan is seeking ways to subvert the Spirit's work of helping people realize their God-given potential. He wants to destroy the temple, the place of honor to God that you are. So the temptations you will face when you diet, and the pain as you begin to get in shape will not be simply the pangs of hunger or the strain of exercise. You may experience the mighty battle between your will and your spirit, the old man and the new man. You may find that you have the desire to do good, but that you cannot carry it out (Romans 7:18). You can say with Paul, "What a wretched man I am! Who will rescue me from this body of death?" (v. 24). You can actually get to that point. You're not just playing for peanuts or calories. You're playing for high stakes in your spiritual life.

But you will also have the grace to cry out, "Thanks be to God—through Jesus Christ our Lord!" (Romans 7:24, 25). You see, God is with you in your weakness, and his power is sufficient to bring you to strength. You may learn through this experience to be dependent upon God for sustenance in a way that you have never known before. He will help you to reach your goal, and will bring you wholeness.

This is where the short-term sense of dieting comes in. Most diets will lay out a menu for a day. Look at it, follow it, but *do not become obsessed with it.* Occupy yourself with something else. Focus on someone else. You must stop thinking about and living for food. Instead, pray that you will live up to your God-given potential—one day at a time.

That's the key—and the way that works best, suggests Overeaters Anonymous. Eat a day, an hour, a minute at a time. Do not worry about tomorrow. Focus on today, how you can follow your regimen immediately, this hour, this minute. And thank God for the discipline.

One of the steps that OA stresses is for us to admit that we are powerless over food. We do not consume food—food consumes us. So we must admit that we are unable to control this urge to eat inappropriately. That might seem impossible, but remember, we became the way we are *because* we did not control the urge to eat.

Another step is to acknowledge our dependence on God for help. Once again, we must admit that we have a problem with food, and that only God can help us solve it.

We also have to be willing to let go of the past, of past failures in dieting or keeping other commitments. We must be willing to accept some risk-taking in order to lose weight *this time*.

We also have to let go of the future. Men are often very results-oriented. We want to know what the outcome of a program will be before we begin. But the end results are actually beyond our control. We can plan sensibly to lose weight, but the success and benefits of the plan are a matter of grace. We must enter into a life-changing process, not only by hard work, but by faith.

A diet can offer an opportunity for us to look within ourselves to see what it is that must be changed in our attitudes. Remember that we are conditioning our minds and spirits as we begin conditioning our bodies and as we diet. We must ask God to forgive us those attitudes which have contributed to our negative self-images. During this time, we also must become aware of how we may have been hurt by others so that food became our friend, our compensation. We must forgive those people, letting go of the hurt they caused us. And we, too, must take a fearless inventory of our own behavior and ask God to heal us of our negativity, despair, and doubt.

Then we must look ahead, to the kind of life we could have as well conditioned, fit people, feeling good inside and outside, and holding healthy attitudes. Think also of a full and fulfilling spiritual life. That full life may be hard to imagine. It was for me. Nonetheless, when I really set my mind to it, I could imagine myself on a beach, running along without a care in the world, free from the shackles of weight and heavy-laden attitudes.

I kept this image before me as I dieted and as I exercised. I must say that, at the end of my regimen, I rewarded myself with a trip to a set of beaches. I felt as whole and complete and healthy as I ever could have imagined myself. So my advice is to try to find a healthy way to treat yourself at the end of your regimen (or as you move to another stage, such as maintenance).

God does give us our heart's desires. If you truly desire to lose weight, and you are willing to examine your heart and mind and soul to ask for healing, then remember that God still has the blueprints for you, and he can still repair and refurbish you.

The construction work is not always easy, however. And from time to time, maintenance repairs have to be made on the temple that you are. The work never stops. But it has to start somewhere. That somewhere, that someone, is you. Today.

FIVE
THE LOSING
BATTLE

The most difficult problem I faced in my journey to physical and spiritual fitness was not temptation while on a diet—although I learned some things I never before knew about temptation. Nor was the problem that I felt physically weak or fatigued during the course of dieting—although I did experience weariness from time to time.

The most difficult problem I faced was admitting that I had both a physical and a spiritual problem, and that I could not solve these problems alone. The hard part for me was to begin, to take action, and to continue in what I knew to be a "losing battle."

"I feel as if I am losing my old self as I watch myself grow thinner," I wrote in an entry in my journal. *"I'm leaving behind an old man with old attitudes. I am becoming a new man. I'm seeing myself and understanding myself, and finding a relationship with God that I've never before known. I'm excited, but I'm also frightened."* I wondered what this new man might be like, how my self-concept and my relationships with others would change. And

yet I was awakening each day with a sense of adventure and exhilaration that I had never known.

My changing attitude and physique were having effects on others as well. Members of the congregation I served would come up to me and say, "There's something about you that's different. You seem filled with new life and energy." Indeed, I did have energy I hadn't known since being a small child. I was hefting less and less weight up and down the flights of stairs to my apartment. I was feeling *good* and eating *good things* for the first time in many years.

I hadn't known what it was like to feel healthy. *"I'm really feeling refreshed as I get out of bed,"* I wrote one day. *"I can't remember ever having a sense of well-being like this. Does obesity really drain one of vitality? I feel not just physical vitality, but spiritual vitality. I am learning more and more how spiritual and physical fitness are brothers."* And on another occasion I wrote, *"I am learning for the first time just how difficult but important discipline is."*

That's one of the primary issues I faced in my life—discipline—although I considered, and do consider, myself to be a disciplined person. During my high school years, I held down a paper route empire, had a public library job, and took extra courses in order to graduate early. I was disciplined in study. During those years I also went to church on a weekly basis. But during my first year of college, I came to know Jesus Christ personally, and asked him into my life to be my Lord and Savior. That was when I learned real spiritual discipline, because

I desired so much to be his servant. I learned something about Bible study, meditation, and the discipline of personal prayer. That kind of discipline is available to anyone who desires to explore more deeply the spiritual life that is awaiting him when he gives himself over to the Lord Jesus Christ.

But I never was able to confront the lack of discipline I had concerning the body God had given me. I could be ordered in so many areas of my life—academic, vocational, even spiritual—but I could not take hold of my appetite. And because I could not get control of that in my life, I was less of a man than I was meant to be. Or *more* of a man, depending on whether you looked within me or outside of me.

What kind of a man can have papers written in advance, keep carefully organized notes, prepare work outlines, organize personal life plans, develop a strategy for a career (originally in law, to which my energies were directed in college), and still have time for a social life—and yet cannot exert self-restraint when it comes to the dinner table? A very hungry man, you say! Nonsense. I was a man who had not come to terms with his principal weakness and asked the Lord to help him deal with it.

I was more than a little smug in self-defense. I had friends in college who had appetites for women, and consumed them like so many sugar cookies. *I was not like* them *in their misconduct!* I told myself. I had a college roommate who had an appetite which I found out later was an addiction to dangerous drugs, and other friends who consumed copious amounts of alcohol. But *I* was not like *them* in their misdeeds. No, I was very moral, very safe in my overeating—or so I thought.

But in my journey to fitness I was confronted with the realization that I was as much a sinner in need of God's grace as were my friends. Perhaps their behavior was more overtly destructive than mine, perhaps easier to condemn. But their sins and mine were identical in source, though not in kind. I finally realized during the days of my rigorous dieting that a trend was developing subtly. Food was close to becoming lord of my life. The power of food for me was overwhelming; to pursue food was to live.

Now, most people cannot understand this passion for food. The ancients called it one of the seven deadly sins: *gluttony.* The word itself *sounds* deadly. The inner attitude is. Gluttony is a serious spiritual issue.

It's interesting to see what the spiritual issues are among those seven sins. They are pride, covetousness, lust, envy, anger, gluttony, and sloth. They all have to do with selfishness and consumption for self. Covetousness is the desire I have to consume my neighbor's goods. Lust is the longing I have to consume another person. Envy is the paralysis that comes over me when I wish I could have what you have. Pride is the paralysis I experience when I build myself up in your eyes, often on information that is not true or at best is manipulated to give you a good impression. Sloth is sheer laziness, my unwillingness to do anything for you or your well-being—or my own, for that matter. Gluttony is the selfish consumption of food.

But what passion is there in pasta? What is so

spiritual about semi-sweet chocolate? Nothing, in itself. It is what my attitude does to food, the way it transforms food that makes it dangerous. The problem is not the *food*. The problem is *me*.

If any one of Jesus' parables speaks to the over-eater, to the "unfit" person—it is the parable of the feeding of the five thousand. Everyone was able to eat and be filled, and the disciples managed to collect twelve baskets of leftover scraps. If I had been there, I could have taken care of another basket, I imagine! All this was accomplished with five loaves of bread and two fishes. Now the people thought that this miracle was so sensational that they tracked Jesus down the next day on the far side of the lake, where he had gone to rest. Jesus told them, "I tell you the truth, you are looking for me, not because you saw miraculous signs but because you ate the loaves and had your fill" (John 6:26). Jesus spoke clearly to the people: *What you're after is a good meal. There's more to life than food!* He said, "Do not work for food that spoils, but for food that endures to eternal life, which the Son of Man will give you" (6:27).

You can have a full stomach, but in pursuit of that full stomach, you can grow spiritually hungry. When you go on a diet, when you consciously seek to challenge your appetites and your habits, you must change your attitude about food and the role it plays in your life. When your belly is not full, or when it is filled with different things at definite times, you begin to sense your spiritual hunger. This spiritual lesson can be most upsetting. It was for me. I was farther from spiritual maturity than I had thought. I discovered the need for discipline in this part of my life which was perhaps the key to becoming a whole, healthy, and happy person in Jesus Christ.

So I listened carefully to his promise. Jesus said, "I am the bread of life. He who comes to me will never go hungry, and he who believes in me will never be thirsty"(John 6:35). Jesus said, *All of your appetites are met in me and me alone.* During the time of my losing battle, I depended more than ever upon the spiritual strength he provided as the Bread of Life. I also held to his words in the Sermon on the Mount in the Gospel according to Matthew. "Therefore I tell you, do not worry about your life, what you will eat or drink; or about your body, what you will wear. Is not life more important than food, and the body more important than clothes?" (Matthew 6:25).

I was caught by that last question: "Is not life more important than food?" In my most honest moments, I had to answer, even with some shame: *No.* Food was more important than life. Not *all* of the time. If it were more important than life all of the time, then I would have been *anorexic,* one who refrains compulsively from eating for fear of being overweight; or I would have been *bulemic,* one who compulsively overeats and then vomits in order not to gain weight. Both are severe psychological and spiritual disorders as well as physical problems. But to me, food was more important than life *some* of the time. That's a spiritual problem.

One danger of dieting I learned is that the dieter can become obsessed with the foods he should and should not be eating. It is as if you put your eating habits under a magnifying glass for a time to determine where the critical fault line is that causes you to desire food to an unhealthy extreme. I followed with rigor the diet that I had chosen and examined carefully what I was eating and how much I was eating of each food, precisely to challenge my habits as well as to lose weight.

Fasting is an altogether different spiritual discipline. To fast is to choose to go *without* food for a time in order to confront your appetites and to provide a space and an openness within, in order to hear God speak. Dieting is a conscious method to lose weight and to change habits permanently. A person who is overweight needs to diet, in my estimation, before choosing to fast. Fasting is a dangerous way to lose weight, and an excellent discipline if you wish to deepen your spiritual life in a significant way.

So I did not fast at any time during my journey to fitness. I needed to learn more about correct and healthy eating patterns before I could actually give up food for a time.

I struggled with dieting a day at a time, trusting God to re-form me into his healthy image. I wrestled with this lack of discipline which dominated other areas of my life and cost me a good deal of money, and potentially my health.

The health club personnel I worked with were very encouraging about prescribing careful exercise during my period of dieting. If your body is accustomed to a greater intake of carbohydrates and sugars, you may feel weary at times, and somewhat weak. Your body is telling you to go slow in your exercise. Gradually, you will be able to build strength and endurance as to the amount of food you allow yourself on your diet, and your body will burn the fat into energy, as a furnace uses fuel that has been stored.

A calorie is an energy unit; 1,800 calories a day will fuel a body to a certain point; then the body has to dip into reserves to convert fat into energy. The more active you are, along with the fewer calories you consume, the more rapid your loss will be. Here's where you have to be careful.

Most doctors recommend that you should lose no more than two pounds a week. Every body is different, and every person's rate of loss differs as a result. But in general, the more slowly the weight comes off, the safer the change is on your system, and the more permanent the loss will be. You see, a body is like a vacuum, in that, when the vacuum is created, something has to fill it to maintain the equilibrium of the system. Weight lost rapidly tends to *return* rapidly, and with a vengeance. So be patient and careful.

And be wise. Do not trust diets which promise that you will lose fourteen pounds in two weeks. I saw one of those ads in a tabloid at the—where else?—supermarket checkout counter. I think it was something like the macaroni, yogurt, and tomato sauce diet. I even hesitate to think about it. Avoid sensational diets. People may push pineapple to excess, then try some other thing like chicken livers the next day, and okra the next. Don't buy a word of it. If it doesn't sound sensible, it probably isn't.

Your body will tell you volumes regarding

whether you're dieting safely. If you feel excessively weak or fatigued for more than a couple of days, if you should notice a change in your heartbeat or blood pressure, or if you feel faint, *check with your physician.* As I said earlier, you need to check with a physician before embarking on a fitness program involving dieting and activity. He or she will be able to guide you safely.

I felt remarkably well during my dieting days—in fact, better than I ever had felt. I was amazed to step on the scale in the morning to see my weight heading slowly but steadily downward. As I continued my circuit training, I could feel myself daily becoming stronger. I began to run regularly as the weather warmed, and I was thrilled to find that I could run at a moderate pace for three miles without being winded. Was God remaking me into an athlete?

As I ran, I envisioned my family cheering me on as I racked up another mile. Soon members of my congregation lined the streets and I imagined myself in some kind of Olympic competition—and not the pie-eating contest! Their encouragement pushed me to extend myself, albeit carefully. Hearing those cheers really lifted my spirits. I guess I forgot to mention what you should do if you're dieting and have hallucinations. . . .

Actually, the *real* support of others became very important to me. I always had been something of an independent guy, as many men are. But I had come up against something that I did not have the willpower to lick by myself. I finally found resolve only because a Christian community cared enough about me to encourage me in a journey to fitness. I was excited, too, to see others in the congregation have the courage to follow my lead, although I didn't feel that I was particularly courageous—I was still rather unsure at that point.

I estimate that, within six months after I began my diet and fitness regimen, the congregation lost over seven hundred pounds. Now that's a successful diet!

I had set my desired goal as 180 pounds. About six weeks into the diet, I arrived at my goal, and I still felt fine. I was wearing new clothes, which gave me a strong impetus to continue carefully to lose weight and to shape up. I continued on the diet for two more weeks and then ate carefully for some weeks afterward. As I continued more and more vigorous exercise (I added aerobic exercise to my regimen), my weight continued to go down as if it were an airliner gliding in for a landing—and not a 747! I passed the 175-pound mark, then 170. Slowly I descended to 165 pounds, and I stayed at that point for an extended period of time.

My body stopped there. I *did* go as low as 158 pounds at one point of extremely vigorous activity (leading a youth group on a mountain retreat; actually, leading a youth group in *anything* physical guarantees weight loss!). I began to become somewhat concerned that I had dipped too low, and for the first time in my life I *had* to eat to gain weight! But not much—I stayed between 163 and 166 pounds for a very long time. Then I went to New Orleans with a friend, ate my way through the French Quarter, and promptly hit 170. I wonder what would happen to a person's weight if he led a youth group to New Orleans. Ah, the perfect maintenance diet! I wouldn't recommend it. New Orleans is a dieter's disaster area.

Our bodies have what is called a "setpoint." That is, you will tend to a certain weight, and a body or physical system will work to stay at that weight. It takes a long time to lower the setpoint once it has been high, but it can be—and has been—done in a careful diet and exercise program. You will know you should stop dieting when, through *sensible* eating patterns and *regular* exercise, your weight remains stable. Mine is about 165 to 170 pounds. It was about 220 to 225 pounds. If you are not careful, you can slowly but surely return to your high setpoint and undo all of the hard work you've put into dieting and exercising for fitness.

I know a woman who must weigh over 200 pounds. She remarked to me one day that I never seemed to gain weight (if only she knew!) and I remained trim. She, on the other hand, could not seem to lose weight, but she also didn't gain more than a pound or two. That's because she has reached her setpoint. Her body will not go above that setpoint except under extraordinary circumstances.

I have a friend, Bill, who nearly ate me out of my summer savings in college as we shared an apartment. Bill was one of those folks who can eat and eat and *never, ever* gain a pound. He was perpetually thin, and he always ate massive portions at dinner, far larger than anything I had. But I gained during that summer! Bill's setpoint was very low, and his metabolism, his use of food consumed, was very high, so he could eat and remain the same weight. I must confess that, during that summer, my self-concept became very low and my envy of him became very high. I had to repent of that memory as I dieted and exercised.

So your body will tell you when you have reached an optimal weight. But you must be careful to stay attuned to your body and not push yourself in your diet beyond what is safe for you. Follow carefully the pattern of the diet. When you are on a stricter portion of the diet, follow it. When you are to maintain, do that. When you reach your goal, then you can evaluate whether or not you wish to continue, or if you now wish to maintain. But listen carefully to your body. Once you remain steady for ten days or more, and you have been dieting carefully and exercising faithfully, you can assume that you have reached your setpoint. Then you should eat carefully and continue your exercise program.

You must also be willing to stop dieting and resume careful, informed, reformed eating habits. You can leave the security of the regimented menus of the diet manual and move out on your own to maintain your newly achieved weight and level of fitness.

I knew I could stop when, one morning, I went with some friends to breakfast—a light one—in a restaurant which has one of those devices for testing your heart rate. They've replaced those old weight-and-fortune machines which always were so embarrassing. A penny could reveal your most closely guarded secret. Now a quarter would reveal one of my cherished revelations. My resting heart rate was in the mid-forties. The average is seventy or so beats per minute. I was beyond average; I was beyond well-conditioned. I was in the athlete range! I really had achieved my goal—a stable and appropriate weight for my build and height, and a good level of fitness in which I felt healthier than I ever could have imagined.

I also felt more fit spiritually. I realized that I truly was free now to work for the food which endures, the food of God's Word and God's service. I was free to be the person I was meant to be, made in God's image. I now was God's temple, honoring him both within and without. I had learned more about the support of the praying and caring Christian community, which had lifted me up as I prayed for strength to deal with gluttony in my own life.

I believe that God can bring any man or woman such a level of discipline in both the physical and the spiritual life. That person simply must be willing to admit that he or she is powerless over food, that food has control over him or her, that food is an idol. Only then can God truly step in to provide the spiritual strength necessary to the achievement of fitness and wholeness.

You must be willing to lose the old self-concepts and the old habits which God wants to break down in you. God seeks to reform and remold you in his image, in wholeness and completeness—in fitness. Fitness for the unfit is a tremendous spiritual struggle which has for its rewards health, vitality, and life.

I frequently had to remind myself just *why* I was exerting all of this effort to lose weight and to grow into fitness. The temptation in our culture, with its concentration on selfishness and ego gratification, is to get into shape *for oneself.* I remember seeing an advertisement for the health club where I was a member. ''I exercise for me,'' beamed a beautiful body from the ad, ''and I love it!''

Now, I do believe that a healthy self-image is very important for a Christian. It reflects something of the beauty of the Holy Spirit at work in a person, helping that person become all that he can be and, I would even say to the overweight person, *less* than he is! But we do not become fit and we do not lose weight as an exercise in self-improvement. If we do, then we face a serious spiritual struggle. God knows that this struggle is ever-present in a secular society where the beautiful person is merely the fit, healthy person. We can make a god out of ourselves and our bodies, with health clubs and jogging tracks becoming the temples and the crystal highways.

I had to resist this temptation to become fit merely as self-improvement. I was following a diet and doing exercise so that I could glorify God in my body, as Paul urges us to do in his first letter to the church in Corinth (1 Corinthians 6:20). I am not my own; I am Christ's, I am God's. So I do not become fit to improve myself. I become fit because, in so doing, I glorify God in my body. I never knew I could do that. Now I know that I *must* do that.

Listen carefully to your body. It will tell you whether what you are doing is sensible as far as diet and exercise are concerned. But listen even more carefully to your body for what it will tell you about the glory of your Creator. And listen to your soul, so that you are not deceived as to the real reason why you fight this losing battle.

As you lose your spiritual and physical insulation, you will hear God speaking to you as you may never before have heard him. You may rely upon him as you never before have relied upon anyone or anything. You will need him as you never have needed anyone or anything else. With God's help, you can win the losing battle.

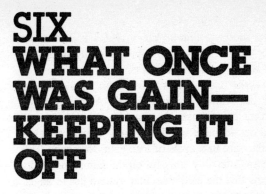

SIX
WHAT ONCE WAS GAIN— KEEPING IT OFF

Recently I read in a newspaper article another of those sad-but-true stories of a person who, heroically, had lost thirty pounds. She kept the weight off for several months. Then she regained fifty-five pounds.

Another person, an acquaintance, went on a liquid protein diet. I saw her after several months, and I almost walked by her without recognizing her. She had lost seventy pounds. She looked wonderful. Recently I saw her again. The tell-tale signs of regaining weight are showing, and she is worried. But she is determined to keep the weight from coming back.

A fellow pastor lost nearly one hundred pounds! He, too, looked and felt fabulous, and he certainly was more vigorous in his ministry as a result of shedding that load. Now he has regained it, and then some. He is mightily discouraged.

A sad fact about weight loss is that, according to one survey, better than 80 percent of those who lose a significant amount of weight will regain it—sometimes more—within a year or two. Put another way, only one out of every five people really finds his or her way to permanent fitness.

Another facet of this figure is not only discouraging, but of great concern as well. A significant percentage of those who regain within a year or two of a considerable weight loss are "repeaters"; that is, they are in a cycle of lose-gain, lose-gain. This pattern is terribly stressful on the human body. It means that the cardiovascular system has to adjust to periods of vigorous exercise, and then periods of none. The system must support a lot of weight, or less weight. And it must accommodate periodic, thorough dieting—which, no matter how sensible and careful it is, always means an alteration in both food intake and food types. The resilient physical body can only take so much. So too with the soul.

Let's look at what the newly-thin person is up against. The successful loser is battling an old setpoint of weight which was very high, and which will tend to return to the setpoint if fitness is not maintained. It takes time for the new setpoint to become established. Then there are old eating patterns which, because of years of habit, are so easy to resume. I *love* chocolate, and I especially enjoy ice cream. Given a choice between a goldbrick sundae and a healthful salad as part of a meal, I will choose the ice cream concoction every time. Now I can— and have—educated myself to enjoy salads, and I do eat and enjoy them. But my ingrained tendency is toward sweets and creams.

I came across a study recently which provided evidence that this tendency to favor sweet things can be traced to infancy. Infants will enjoy a sweet food, such as fruit, and choose it more often than a food with a bitter or sharp taste. That's why parents must be especially careful to give their children a well-balanced diet that goes easy on the sweets. And I have learned the hard way that sweets must *never* be used as a reward for doing something good. I would hate to count how many times I have stopped for a sundae on my way somewhere. When you consider yourself a good person, you can really pay a price!

So newly fit people tend to return to the habits with which they are familiar, which have brought them comfort, security, and enjoyment for many years. On the other hand, the tendency to avoid exertion, to live at ease, is also branded deeply within the overweight person. There are always many more good reasons to miss a period of exercise during the day than to miss a meal or to pass up a snack. One can usually get a meal on the run from a fast-food palace and return to the duties of the day in no time flat. Taking off for exercise does involve a chunk of time which many of us find difficult to carve out of our busy schedules.

Then there are those people who meet you and think that you've *always* been thin, and ask you how *they* can get that way—as they offer you a piece of pie or another helping of lasagna. Turning down food is for me one of the most difficult necessities of life. I think of eating together, and sharing someone else's bread, to be at times a holy act. People have often made great efforts to set a lovely meal before me. I am almost contemptuous of their gift if I turn down such a meal, or so I feel. Here's another example of how guilt and eating are so often tied together. I feel guilty if I say no to an offer of food. *She worked so hard to prepare the food. It will go to waste if I don't have it. It will turn into leftovers, and he'll have to endure it.* These are but three thoughts that go through my mind as I struggle with those who push food on me. I let them do it, I feel bad about refusing, and I feel worse within if I eat it. I picture those happy little fat cells in my body just loving every morsel that comes their way. So I have to say no in as graceful and positive a way as I know how, and be able to take responsibility for my own actions.

The pitfalls to maintaining a desired weight and fitness, then, are many and varied. It is no wonder that, for so many, the weight comes pouring back within a short time. Even the strongest person finds that maintenance is difficult at best. Christians are not immune to these trials—and trials they are, because the problem is not merely physical, but deeply spiritual, as we have seen. But does the Christian have access to some greater healing power which transforms the will, the source of the problem for many who suffer from obesity? Some people— relatively few—do have a medical problem of obesity, and they have access to medication and monitoring to help them maintain a balanced weight. But most of us—perhaps all of us—who struggle with overeating have to grapple with the spiritual problem and accept the spiritual solution.

The Christian remembers that Jesus Christ suffered in life because he, too, was tempted. So he is able to help those who are undergoing temptation

(Hebrews 2:18). He was tempted in every way that we are, yet he did not sin (4:15). So the Christian can pray with confidence to God through Jesus Christ in the midst of temptation and challenge to discipline and say, "Lord, help me. I cannot overcome this temptation by myself." We are human beings, and we will sin. We will succumb to culinary (and other) temptations. If we do, we should be careful not to blame ourselves excessively, but we must be able to admit our wrongs, remember that we really are powerless when it comes to food, and start over again.

I came to a time in my life when I could enjoy a good and healthy meal, and I could see my favorite sweet as a treat, not as a necessity. Generally, it is a good thing not to have these items of temptation around the house. With a family, the temptations are usually there and they are difficult to resist. It is likely that your wife and children too could stand to eat more carefully and avoid certain rich foods. But it may not be fair to impose your discipline on them unless they choose to support you—and I would hope that they do. Just make it a habit to stay out of range of the refrigerator, and to be active and choose to do things, more and more, which you do *not* associate with food.

I learned to savor those foods which formerly I had consumed quickly. I was surprised to learn that I really had not enjoyed them before because I had not taken the time to appreciate them. But I could now begin to taste them once in a while, a little at a time, and know that I had set a stopping point. This is another key to maintaining weight: set limits. I will have that forbidden food, but only in this amount, and only with such and such a frequency. I limited my ice cream to a scoop a week. I looked forward to that scoop and was satisfied with it.

I also exercised it off. Here is where diet and exercise truly are a pair. I kept to a regular schedule of exercise, with variety both indoor and outdoor, every day of the week. I arranged to meet friends at the health club or on a jog, rather than at the restaurant for lunch. I can even recall a couple of very interesting occasions of counseling with a parishioner while we both were out running.

I knew that I could eat a certain quantity, exercise a given amount, and remain stable in weight. I learned just what I could eat and how much activity I needed in order to maintain. I can't say that I was very scientific about the whole procedure. I had more of an intuitive knowledge of what eating and exercise patterns worked for me. As my level of exercise became more vigorous, and as I finished my diet, I was astonished to discover one day that I really wasn't "hungry" or seeking food—and that I hadn't wanted much to eat in days. Formerly, that would have been a sign of certain illness; now it was a sign of certain health. And when I ate, I didn't want much—and this from the second-helping champion! Others who had dieted successfully reported to me the same phenomenon. At the end, we neither felt hungry nor thought about food, and one fact supported the other. Plus we loved to exercise.

Exercising also helped me to control some of the stress which had given me a good excuse to eat. In reaction to confrontation, human beings usually exhibit a fight-or-flight reaction. I had an eat reaction—a form of flight, I suppose. I never could fly very high—perhaps like a penguin.

In the ministry, there are always things that you want to say to people—or sometimes that you even would like to *do* to them—when they level an unfair criticism at you, say a most cutting thing, or simply act irresponsibly. Any businessman can identify with the situation. In a pastor's work there are people to manage, people for whom you care. And if you have the least amount of compassion as a pastor, the pains and losses of your own parishioners become yours, too. More stress, more conditioned response: eat.

Exercise has a marvelous effect on stress. It works it away. It is as though stress stokes the fires of exercise. Perhaps it is the fuel of fitness. A pastor and friend of mine says that he goes running to ease the stress he feels. Believe me, at that rate, I could keep the shoe industry humming with the running I should be doing! Another pastor—I kid you not—has punching bags in his garage. He comes home from the office or from visitations and *WHAM! WHAM! WHAM!* One for Mrs. Smith's complaint about the tulips around the church being the wrong color. *WHAM!* One for the chairman of the church board's half-hour argument with other board members about $12.00 a year savings by using single-fold instead of double-fold paper towels. *WHAM!* There's one for the new denominational requirement of a 50 percent growth in membership for his church next year. *WHAM!* Afterward, does he feel relaxed! His wife must think that he has an easy job as he comes in from the garage, tranquil after a long day of work.

When church members anger me—and from time to time they do—or when I get riled up about denominational politics, I find that I run my best times, and my longest distances. What a healthy way to work off stress. The time spent away from the situation, away from the phone—fresh air, the total use of the body—all combine to give me a better perspective when I return to the fray. I also burn up the calories and keep the weight down.

It is important to establish some kind of routine. If you are self-employed, as a pastor is, you must have the discipline and freedom to develop an exercise schedule. If you work for someone else, you may have to work your routine around your office responsibilities. Some companies have begun to recognize the benefits they receive from promoting and encouraging health among their employees. A member of a church I pastored was the personnel director for a major national food producer. In their gleaming new headquarters building was a fully equipped and staffed workout center. People were given some time each day to use the facilities, which were part of the salary and benefit package. Other companies will pay for club memberships for their employees, realizing that exercise and proper diet make for a more productive and vigorous employee. Would that all church boards understood this principle also, and encouraged their pastors to stay in shape!

One can travel now and stay in hotels in major cities which provide health clubs and spa facilities.

Some even have jogging tracks, and others will provide maps of their area with preferred routes plotted out for the cosmopolitan runner. So even those workers for whom travel is a way of life can remain fit.

The greatest challenge to my fitness came when I changed churches and moved. Any change in life—a move, the birth of a child, the death of a loved one, the beginning of a new job—can mean disruption of a carefully worked out routine, or loss of familiar clubs or running routes. You may move away from encouraging friends who have been willing to work out with you, and people who have known you both overweight and thin.

I have struggled personally with maintenance of my weight for several years, so I know what a challenge it can be. I married, moved, and started a new job as pastor all within three months. In a little over a year's time, our first child was born. By my calculations, I should be over 500 pounds! Seriously, I do battle to maintain my weight and level of fitness. I don't think one ever stops having to do that.

But the maintenance of a balanced life is always a process. One never finds perfect stasis. Yet the best way to begin is through inner discipline. It is important that you and I understand ourselves *holistically.* That is, we see ourselves as whole persons, with the diverse components of our lives drawn into unity by the Holy Spirit. As human beings, we are physical, emotional, spiritual, and intellectual. When one part falls out of balance with the others, we feel it in all areas. Undue stress in one area has an effect on us as whole persons. Strengthening ourselves in one area touches all the other points.

I always thought that my intellectual life was separate altogether. But I discovered that how I *thought* about myself was indeed how I *felt* about myself—which influenced the way I *perceived* myself, which also affected my weight. You cannot simply aim to change one area in your life without experiencing shock waves. So when you make an effort to discipline one area of your life, the other parts of your life may reveal further needs for discipline. It takes courage to disrupt your present situation and risk facing a major life overhaul!

How can you ever get "in balance"? Just as you balance your checkbook to see how much money you have available to you, you need to balance your time to discover how much you have to use, what things you need to do, and which people you need to see. You need to balance your meals, to be sure that you are getting what you need of the right things. These four areas of your life—physical, spiritual, emotional, and intellectual—all require work to get all you can out of what God has given you. You can be balanced, you can be disciplined, with practice and responsibility on your part, and with the help of the Holy Spirit ordering your unruly will.

There are several things you can do to help achieve the balance you need to maintain your good weight and newfound fitness:

First, set a goal. For example, decide that you want a stable weight of, say, 170 pounds (if you are a 6'0" male) for six months. Then, having accomplished this goal, set it for another six months—and so on. Actually, you may have to set out to do this by the day, or the week. Gradually, you will continuously maintain your weight.

Second, prepare to enter a competition—not with the intent to win a prize, but rather to train to the best of your ability. Every year there is a 10-kilometer run in my neighborhood which I think is the best in the city—our area has lots of hills, a runner's paradise. So I train for that to compete only against myself. The training by itself is a valuable experience.

Third, plan your meals. Know what you want to eat and when you want to eat it. Shop ahead. Shopping at the supermarket just before dinner when I am very hungry is usually disastrous for me.

Plan your treats. It's all right to have a treat from time to time—and even better to plan ahead so that you can look forward to it and you won't be tempted to splurge just any time.

Fourth, make an appointment to exercise—just as you would to have lunch with a client, or sit down to discuss your work with your secretary. Put your exercise time on your calendar in pen, and do not move it unless absolutely necessary.

Fifth, balance your day with some spiritual preparation which will help to put your dieting and exercise into perspective, and relieve you of some of your anxieties. One of the most helpful books is the daily meditation *Food for Thought* (Hazelden), which is used by many chapters of Overeaters Anonymous. OA uses the Twelve Step Method that has been developed with such success by Alcoholics Anonymous. They also use the "serenity prayer": "Lord, grant me the serenity to accept the things I cannot change, the courage to change the things I can, and the wisdom to know the difference." And just as AA urges its members to think one day at a time, so should you—even one meal at a time, if necessary.

Should you need additional support from other people in your new eating habits, why not participate in Overeaters Anonymous? There are thousands of chapters all across the United States, in large cities and small towns. Look in the phone book to learn how to find the chapter nearest you. Your local hospital, or possibly your pastor, might be able to refer you to a chapter.

These all are ways in which you can maintain your newfound weight level and fitness. The secret is balance. It is the gift of God as well as the responsibility of human beings. One day you will come to the point where food does not matter much anymore, and when you effortlessly enjoy your exercise. The day will come for you, if you are patient, persistent, and purposeful.

SEVEN
FOOD FOR
THOUGHT

The diet book is probably America's principal
growth industry. As I was doing some background
work for this book, I looked through the card
catalog at the Chicago Public Library and counted
close to 130 diet books in the file. Perhaps there
were even more lurking under other categories:
FOOD, Love of; or, CAUSES, Hopeless. More
books are coming out each month on the subject,
each with extravagant claims which can lure the
gullible into nutritional disaster.

How do you choose a diet book? A fitness book? I
remember going into a major bookstore to look for a
diet plan and staring at the array of names and
claims. I skimmed several books. I asked friends
what had worked for them—word of mouth is
perhaps the most trustworthy recommendation. Did I
ask my doctor? No, but then, as I have said, he
wasn't very helpful in nutritional matters. Today
more doctors are becoming better informed on the
subject, and some are willing to work in conjunction
with a nutritionist. But I chose my diet without any

real help from anyone. I am grateful that the diet did not do any damage to me, and I am glad that I continued to exercise vigorously. One must be exceedingly careful in choosing a diet. And it is best to see the diet, along with the exercise, as means to an end—of better eating habits and overall fitness.

A diet is not worth the paper it's printed on if it does not change *both* your cooking *and* your eating habits. And in order for the diet truly to be effective, you must exercise regularly as part of your newfound discipline. Now I want to say a word about those advertisements for gizmos which promise that you will lose so many pounds per day as you lounge around your house. If losing weight were that easy, then a lot of people would be much thinner than they are! The principle is that the heat generated from these garments, or the "massage" from exercise units, will literally melt off the pounds as though you were a tub of butter.

Actually, what is happening, if anything, is that you are experiencing water loss, which will show up as weight loss on the scale. The same thing happens after you have been exercising on a warm day and perspiring profusely. The body will see to it that this liquid is replaced when you drink two or three glasses of water, as you should—and more—each day. Thus the weight returns. With these gizmos you have experienced no cardiovascular benefits from any exercise, and you have not burned off any "fat deposits." You have been taken instead.

Such items appeal to the overweight person's intense desire to make taking weight off as easy as it was to put on, and as pleasurable. Now, I happen to think that a good run, or a weight training circuit, is very pleasurable; but it certainly wasn't at first. If you seek a life of ease, then a diet and exercise program will discourage you. But remember: No effort, no loss.

Your habits must change. It's as simple as that. But how we fight those changes of habit, even when we know they are for the better! "I do not understand what I do," says the apostle Paul. "For what I want to do I do not do, but what I hate I do. . . . I have the desire to do what is good, but I cannot carry it out. For what I do is not the good I want to do; no, the evil I do not want to do—this I keep on doing" (Romans 7:15, 18b, 19). This could be the overweight person's lament as he approaches a diet. And he is always trying to find an easy way out.

So if it isn't gimmicks in equipment, then it is a gimmick in a diet. I had a professor in seminary who, from time to time, sought to lose weight. She claimed that for one day she ate only ice cream, and she lost weight. Thus was born the Edna Evans Miracle Ice Cream Diet which, were it true, would have found me as its first experimental subject! But one look at the variety of diets will reveal that gimmicks are too often the word of the day for them, and the gimmicks are dangerous. Dr. Charles Kuntzleman in his *No-Diet Fitness Book* (Tyndale House, 1984), has a very helpful chart on diets which I recommend you review before you venture into the dieting world. There are six dieting categories, according to his research: low-carbohydrate diets, low-fat diets, high carbohydrate diets, high-fat diets (see how contradictory so many dieting theories

are!); high protein diets; and other diets, including
liquid diets, the latest rage. Dr. Kuntzleman reviews
the diet claims of each and then makes a medical
analysis of those claims, and predicts the likely
results of those diets. His chart is most revealing.
My choice, which was the Scarsdale Diet, doesn't
fare too well. As a low-carbohydrate diet, it scores
low because most of the weight loss is water, kidney
function is stressfully increased, and it lacks vitamins
and minerals that a balanced diet provides. Fatigue is
a common and real problem, as well, because of the
lack of carbohydrates.

Carbohydrates are a primary source of energy.
Some are simple carbohydrates, often found in junk
food or sweets—and they are high in calories and
fat, which make for nutritional nonsense. Complex
carbohydrates are found in fruits, legumes, pasta,
and grains, and they sometimes are very low in
calories. They provide a wide range of energy and
nutrition to many parts of the body.

You can consult Dr. Kuntzleman's chart for
specific details regarding diets. He and I agreed on
three things: First, you must reduce your caloric
intake, for that is where the excess pounds add on.
What difference does it make, strictly speaking, if
you eat 2,000 calories worth of ice cream or the
same caloric amount of, say, squash? I'll tell you
one thing—you'd enjoy the ice cream a lot more, if
you're like me! So look for a *well-balanced* diet that
is low in calories. You will follow some diet—that
is, a way of eating—all of your life in order to stay
within a reasonable weight range. So you should
look for one with balance.

Second, as I've said again and again, I have learned that a diet is absolutely worthless without exercise. As you reduce your caloric intake, you should work on cleaning out your calorie warehouse—all those calories you've carefully stored for years. Fitness is the simple equation: a sensible diet plus sensible exercise.

Third, look deep within you for the spiritual problem that may be at the root of your weight problem. Do a spiritual inventory. Again, there are those who for medical reasons cannot easily maintain reasonable body weight, and there are some who seem to have something in their genetic makeup that predisposes them to obesity. Yet these problems too may have spiritual ramifications.

I might add, too, that it is important to reeducate yourself about food. I was surprised that, while I enjoyed food so much and cooked it well, I really didn't know much about sensible nutrition—how foods worked with the body. Maybe I was asleep in biology class, but I don't remember ever having been taught much on the subject. Perhaps nutritional management would be a good thing to teach in our schools as a practical science where the Potato Chip and Brownie Diet seems to reign. Add those poor choices to the perils of institutional cooking and you have disaster. One evening in college I was standing in the cafeteria line only to discover that supper was—I am dead serious—*liver creole* and something called *cheese dreams* (nightmares, to be sure). Suddenly a potato chip and brownie diet looks *very* good.

Diet for a Small Planet by Frances Moore Lappe

was an important educational tool for me as I began learning about food, nutritional chains within the body, and food chains on planet Earth. We Americans are sometimes very poor stewards of food. We may eat too much of the wrong thing. It is only because we do eat *so much*—as much as 2,000 pounds of food a year—that we manage to find all of the nutrients we need, often by mistake or unintentionally. People in Third World areas eat much less than we do, but manage to get their nutrients much more efficiently. Of course, in the areas where famine is the order of the day, neither food nor nutrients reach people. That should spur us on to more awareness of what we waste—as well as what we eat, why we eat it, and what we *should* be eating for health's sake. As world citizens and stewards of God's creation we also need to educate ourselves and evaluate our responsibilities toward the other people who share our planet.

So, for me, a diet was not an end in itself, but rather the means by which I could learn more about what I was consuming and why—to become, in a word, an *informed* consumer. I have come to eat much less red meat than I formerly did, and to begin to eat more complex carbohydrate meals. Perhaps that's how the Irish have managed to get by on their potatoes and the Italians on their pasta. Concentrated proteins, such as fish, are also a good source in the food chain. As I say, I allow myself sweets. But I always try to eat them moderately and then exercise them off. I strive for a reasonable balance.

The May 31, 1983, *Family Circle* has a little section which I have found helpful in determining what makes a good diet. Gradual, steady weight loss is important—beware of extravagant promises. There should also be a balance of nutrients: 20 percent protein, 30 percent fat, and 50 percent carbohydrate. That is the optimal balance for fueling the body for the other component of the good diet: exercise.

What is the best overall exercise you can do? Walking. That's all—good, *vigorous* walking for at least twenty minutes. The romantic saunter on the beach won't do, I'm afraid, though it might cause other chemical processes to heat up in the body. But that's another story. Walking requires no special equipment, it does not cost very much, if anything, to begin—although you will want a comfortable pair of shoes. And you can do it in any season, in almost any weather. Walking is the no-excuse exercise, perfect for sedentary eaters as they begin their quest for fitness.

Of course, depending on where you live, you may not be able to walk anywhere just any time you choose. I wouldn't recommend walking in Central Park or in other crime-ridden areas late at night; use common sense. Of course, you could get into trouble in the suburbs, too. Not all that long ago, a minister and a friend were walking in a suburb when a policeman spotted them, pulled up, ordered them up against the squad car, and began to question them. *No one* walked in that suburb; therefore, he figured they were suspicious characters!

But that's not too likely to happen in fitness-conscious America. Walking is a good choice for basic exercise to accompany a new eating plan.

I chose circuit-training—timed, vigorous, repetitive

activity guaranteed to use up a lot of calories. Much, much later I began weight training to firm up in the areas where I had slimmed down. Pastor Schwarzenegger I'm not; I'm not a bodybuilder by any means—I would have been condemned long ago for sagging foundations! However, I did find that this activity, combined with aerobic dance under careful supervision, helped me to maintain a stable weight.

I ran. I did not jog, I ran. A jog is a slow-paced effort, or perhaps running at a relaxed level. I gradually tried to build up speed and endurance so that I could cover a lot of ground quickly. I also was *very* careful to warm up and cool down properly before running or doing any aerobic activity. If you take up running you must be careful to do the same. It will help you to avoid injury and will make the most of your fitness efforts.

As I think about my time in circuit training, I realize that I had an unusually positive experience with a health club. You can, too, if you follow certain guidelines. I was on my lunch hour when I made my initial visit to the health club. That was generally when I planned to be there, so I had a good idea of the number of people using the equipment at that hour, the wait between stations, the quality of supervision, and the crowd in the locker room. At that time of day I experienced a very positive attitude toward the facilities. Had I gone there regularly at 5:30 P.M. on a weeknight, I probably would have wondered if I were in the same club, the crush of people could be so oppressive.

I was interviewed by an instructor who treated me as a person, offering me a service which could improve my well-being. He did not approach me with dollar signs in his eyes, viewing me merely as another sale. He took time to explain the program, determine my physical condition, show me the circuit, and demonstrate the equipment. You should be wary of anyone who does not take that kind of time. If you are as ignorant as I was of the equipment, you could do yourself great physical harm if you are not shown the right technique. At best, your efforts could be worthless—you could be doing the exercise all wrong.

Read your contract carefully. I knew that once I plunked down my entrance fee and first month's payment, I was in for good. I didn't *want* out of the contract. But some people do change their minds and discover that they cannot get out of the contract as easily as they got in. Read the terms carefully and be sure that you want that kind of discipline. Some clubs offer a short-term membership or a fee-for-use plan in the event that you do not want to work out every day.

The YMCA or YWCA is a good alternative to the private health club with its naked profit motive for your improved physique. The Y may not be as fancy and colorful as the deluxe models, but as a generic health club, it will offer everything you need. Dan Baum of the *Wall Street Journal* (January 18, 1985) also suggests that you can sometimes gain access to university facilities by taking a night class, for which you will obtain an I.D. Sometimes a university will offer use of its facilities for nonstudents at a special fee. You only need ask. Wherever you go, make sure the staff is trained, especially if you're just starting out in the world of exercise.

The problem with buying your own home gym center is that, if you are not very knowledgeable about fitness and exercise, you could risk injury. On the other hand, these home centers offer convenience that is unmatched. (No excuses, either, in any weather!) You can exercise at any hour of the day or night. Most of all, no one has to see your hefty frame wrestle in a life-or-death manner with a torturous machine. It will behoove you to *read, read, read* all you can about exercise equipment before you buy so that you get exactly what you want and need. Any salesperson will be more than eager to sell you an entire system which will cost you an arm and a leg, fit or unfit, if that's what you want. So *know what you want,* and find a shop where the staff doesn't look like they just came from the donut shop.

Doing exercises to records, cassettes, and videos doesn't do much for me; and, as a result, I don't do much for them. I've long thought that these videos were a means for displaying how certain human beings are actually made out of play-dough. I mean, how many of us can *really* contort like that? And is that fitness? Does it improve the cardiovascular system? And will you risk injury because of some celebrity's strange notions of good exercise? Anyway, with the use of media, you do not have the benefit of a trained individual who can monitor your workout and correct what you're doing wrong. That is vitally important as you begin your discipline of exercise.

Perhaps you find fitness is more pleasurable in

numbers. I liked to work out with others, although basically I am a solo runner. While I'm running I gather my thoughts, or think about nothing at all, but listen to birds singing, the wind blowing through the trees, or the rhythm of my own heartbeat. That is a very holy time for me, and a time I generally do not want to share with others, unless I have a very understanding and quiet partner. On the other hand, to run or walk or work out with others means that you can't weasel out of the commitment simply because you feel lazy. After all, that other person is counting on you.

I must admit that I have carried to an extreme working out with others. One Sunday morning I climbed into my pulpit and opened with prayer just after people had concluded singing a hymn. As I concluded my prayer, I asked everyone to remain standing. I then had everyone do stretching exercises in the pews. I resisted the urge to begin barking a count for calisthenics. Now, this church building had a round chancel area. Can you picture an entire congregation doing forty laps around the church as an object lesson on "Strengthening Your Faith"? I didn't do it, but it was one of those great living illustrations which people surely would have remembered had they survived it.

The greatest fitness effort that the congregation ever did undertake was in golf—an exercise of dubious fitness value unless you walk the course. Even so, it's not the express lane to fitness. At the congregational golf tournament one time I was awarded the Bent Shaft for the highest score ever achieved in one game. It's a mystery to me why I manage to gain the highest scores in sports requiring low scores, and low scores in high-scoring competitions! I may be a fitness enthusiast, but I'm not much of a sportsman. Fortunately, you don't have to be a sportsman to be in shape. You simply have to be wise in your choice of exercise.

I was heartened by the thorough support those members of the congregation gave me, as the numbers on my scale decreased. Do not hesitate to share with others your weight loss efforts. Tell those who are interested some of the details of your diet and exercise program so that they will know specifically how to support you and pray for you. It's amazing how people will give you verbal encouragement, or practical help such as sharing low-calorie recipes.

Next to my French-cooking classics in my kitchen are several low-cal cookbooks. The *Weight-Watchers 365-Day Cookbook* is very good, offering great balance in nutrients and good variety in food types. As I eliminated butter and salt from most foods at the table and in preparation, I was reminded just how *good* good food tastes. I lightened up sauces, poached foods such as fish, and steamed vegetables. I moved away from processed foods and frozen entrees, which are generally brimming with salt or sugar and fat. I am encouraged by the new lighter meals now available in the frozen food case. But I prefer my own cooking in which I can determine to a large extent how much of what goes into the preparation. Spices have taken the place of salt and butter in many dishes. For a diet to work in the long run, *you must learn to cook differently.*

You must also be careful in restaurants. So many places serve enough food to supply a Roman army on campaign for months. The amounts piled on plates can be obscene at times. Salad bars can be dangerous, especially when you dig into the cream-laden potato salad. Stick to spinach and lettuce, and garnish with a prudent selection of fresh fruit. And eat adequately. I must admit that I still feel a tinge of guilt when I do not clean my plate. But I am trying to learn to ask for a person-bag (I don't have a dog, and most dogs could stand a little weight control anyway!) so that I can enjoy my unfinished entree at another time. Go easy on the bread and butter, too. Do I sound more and more like your mother? Sorry. Just one more thing—eat slowly and *chew* your food. I used to swallow food almost whole without taking time to chew, thus missing the very enjoyment for which I longed when I would eat! I needed to slow down the eating process. I enjoy Chinese cuisine, and I have learned to manipulate chopsticks, which forces me to eat more slowly and with greater concentration and care.

OK, I *am* your mother for one more minute. If you shop, as I do, for the family, go *after* mealtime. Shopping on an empty stomach is like letting locusts loose on a ripe grain field. If I go before lunch, I buy like I'm a contestant on Supermarket Sweep. I always grab things I don't need, really don't want, and shouldn't eat. Plan your meals and plan your shopping to buy what you really need rather than what you think you need or wish you could eat.

Changing your eating habits is an important part of successful dieting. A sensible diet is a pattern of good eating throughout your life. It is elemental, along with exercise to attain fitness. To support your change in eating habits, you must also change your cooking and your shopping habits. That takes education in nutrition, which is essential to eating wisely and living healthfully. Take time to learn about what you eat so that you can make wise choices.

Make wise choices, too, about your exercise program. Read carefully and list your options, especially when it comes to joining a health club and spending money doing so. Know what you want to accomplish *before* you begin. Be observant of claims which cannot be fulfilled or of staff which is not attentive. You want to go where you will be led into fitness, not fall into it by neglect.

Finally, let other people support you in your efforts in fitness. You cannot do it alone. You need others who can encourage you, lead you, help you, and talk with you. You also need someone who can pray with you about the spiritual dimensions of your struggle to become fit and to enter a new phase of life. You need someone who can truly give you food for thought.

EIGHT
EXERCISING
YOUR FAITH

Of all people, Christians should be the advocates of a healthy life style. Christians realize that God has blessed them with a body which, as David says, is "fearfully and wonderfully made" (Psalm 139:14). The human body is the penultimate creation of God—next to the soul. With the body we can glorify God, praising him fully through physical means. The apostle Paul urges the Christians at Rome, "in view of God's mercy, to offer your bodies as living sacrifices, holy and pleasing to God—which is your spiritual worship" (Romans 12:1). He tells the Corinthians, "You are not your own; you were bought at a price. Therefore honor God with your body" (1 Corinthians 6:19b, 20).

Paul, a good Jewish theologian who met the Lord and surrendered his life to the Lord's service, never lost the Jewish understanding that there was no distinction between the spirit (or the mind) and the body, the physical creation of God. The Greeks clearly differentiated between body and spirit, lifting up the spirit, the mind, over the body (which was, in their thinking, of little account). We are heirs to this way of thinking and believing. Thus we assume that how we use our bodies and what we think with our minds are two entirely different things.

The Jewish understanding, which was brought into the Christian faith, is a much healthier view of human life in all its fullness. It assumes that our physical beings and our spiritual persons are intimately linked. Of course, we experience inner conflicts, particularly as we confront our various appetites. But by the power of the Holy Spirit, we can have victory over those impulses which make for unhealthful living, living without fitness.

Paul says, "live by the Spirit, and you will not gratify the desires of the sinful nature" (Galatians 5:16). A major problem in American culture, in which each of us shares, Christian or non-Christian, is the desire for gratification. A college friend of mine found the perfect slogan to describe our age: "I want it all, and I want it now." To diet, to engage in exercise, to seek fitness, is to work contrary to the desire for gratification. We want to fulfill those desires of our sinful natures. But gratification is not God's way. Blessing is. And fitness is a blessing from God, who rewards our efforts, strengthens our resolve, and prospers our responsibilities. But this blessing from God is not easy to receive.

Paul continues, "For the sinful nature desires what is contrary to the Spirit, and the Spirit what is contrary to the sinful nature. They are in conflict with each other, so that you do not do what you want" (Galatians 5:17). But through God's help, by the power of the Holy Spirit, you can overcome any lack of will. Yet at the same time, you must be responsible for your action—or inaction—in diet and exercise. You could say that God lets you work out your own fitness in fear and trembling. And sometimes in exhaustion. Fitness is not easy to attain or maintain—but it is necessary.

If it were easy, then we could use spiritual sauna belts to lose weight and become fit. We would innately want to eat what is good for us. But the truth, as I know, and as you know, too, is that we do not make those healthful choices. We seek to be sedentary, not only physically, but spiritually as well. I'm just waiting for someone to write a book, *Flattening Your Stomach Through Prayer.* If only that were possible, there would be so much prayer power, not only as to remove mountains, but to shed pounds. I sometimes think that the latter would be harder.

What we seek is self-control, which, Paul says, is a *fruit of the Spirit,* a result of the Holy Spirit at work in the believer. "Those who belong to Christ Jesus have crucified the sinful nature with its passions and desires," Paul says. So, "Since we live by the Spirit, let us keep in step with the Spirit" (Galatians 5:24, 25). Paul is calling us to exercise our faith as we strive for fitness.

We seek self-control, not gratification. That is the Christian's goal of fitness, another way by which we are being made perfect for God through our Lord Jesus Christ. We realize that the ultimate goal of the right use of our bodies is not to glorify ourselves in this life, but to testify to God's presence in us as long as we are alive. We want to exemplify that fitness that is within our hearts and minds and which shows forth in our physical bodies. But physical fitness is not the ultimate end we seek. It is wholeness—full human fitness as one of God's creatures.

That's what Paul means when he says that the human body is actually decaying in this life. You might well live longer and healthier with a better outlook and a deeper view of life. But even fit people die. Jim Fixx, the great runner, who himself was an overweight, out-of-shape man for many years, discovered fitness fairly late in his tragically shortened life. He became a marathon runner, taught fitness, exuded well-being. Yet he died at age fifty-two of a heart attack while running before an appearance at a seminar. Coronary blockage seemed to run in his family. His grandfather and father had both died at tragically young ages.

Jim Fixx probably would have joined their ranks at a much earlier age had he not become a strong and fit individual. Some medical experts figure that he lived nearly ten years longer because he was in such good shape. But even fit people die—not because of their fitness or their diet or exercise in itself. Fit people die because all people die. If you hoped that you would find immortality through fitness, you can forget it. But you can make the most of the life you are given as a fit and healthy person.

Paul says, "Though outwardly we are wasting away, yet inwardly we are being renewed day by day. For our light and momentary troubles are achieving for us an eternal glory that far outweighs them all. So we fix our eyes not on what is seen,

but on what is unseen. For what is seen is temporary, but what is unseen is eternal'' (2 Corinthians
4:16b-18). You'll find your glory in another life.
But you and I are to glorify God as best we can in
this life, by being good stewards of the marvelous
physical house which he has given us. We are called
to become a temple in which he dwells.

So as you and I seek to be fit Christians, not fat
Christians, we must always remember *why* we seek
fitness. The reasons are not only personal, not only
physical; they are spiritual in nature as well. We
glorify God with the best minds we can be, the best
bodies we can develop, and the strongest spiritual
people we can become. It is God's work in us. The
keys to this unity of fitness are *balance* and
discipline, and we never stop learning how to be
balanced and disciplined in our lives. But that is
what God wants, and he will help us to become
those things.

We are always more than we appear to be, if we
accept the reality of our spiritual nature. In the end,
we will be more than we ever dreamed we could be.
Fitness is just a taste of the personal wholeness
which God has promised every believer, to be discovered in the resurrection. God cares for bodies.
That is part of the mystery of the Incarnation, God
taking human flesh, a *body,* in Jesus Christ. That is
also part of the meaning of the resurrection, wherein
God raised much more than human spirit; he raised
Jesus' *body,* and it was more wonderful than anyone
could attempt to describe. We, too, will be fit and
whole beyond anything we can accomplish or imagine in this life when we consider that our bodies,

too, will be raised at the last day. Paul says, "The body that is sown [in human life] is perishable, it is raised imperishable; it is sown in dishonor, it is raised in glory; it is sown in weakness, it is raised in power; it is sown a natural body, it is raised a spiritual body" (1 Corinthians 15:42b-44a).

So we focus on fitness because it is a foretaste of the life to come, life in wholeness of fellowship with God. We are privileged to have some sense of what risen life will be like as we experience a healthy and fit life here on earth day by day. We have been given a body with which to work, the food with which to fuel fitness, a will being disciplined by the Holy Spirit, and an understanding of why fitness is so important in God's plan for human life. Christians are fit, not because it is in fashion (it hasn't always been), not because we gratify our desires or glorify ourselves, but because God would have us be that way.

But we must be at work. We must be in training for total fitness as Christians. Paul, that champion of examples of the body and the relation of physical and spiritual life, gives us another example of the training ahead of us. "Do you not know that in a race all the runners run, but only one gets the prize? Run in such a way as to get the prize" (1 Corinthians 9:24). The Christian life frequently is described in terms of physical training and discipline: *walk* in the Spirit, *walk* in love, *walk* in the way, *run, train,* and so forth. "Everyone who competes in the games goes into strict training," Paul continues. "They do it to get a crown that will not last;

but we do it to get a crown that will last for ever''
(1 Corinthians 9:25).

Athletes who train for the Olympic games give up
a portion of their lives to be able to participate in
this competition which pits the finest, fittest men and
women of the world against one another. They enter
the strictest training imaginable so as to achieve the
ultimate level of fitness possible. They work hard at
this to bring glory, not so much to themselves as to
their country and their people. These courageous
men and women adhere to very strict diets, careful
mental and emotional preparation to withstand the
strains of competition, and rigorous, consistent
physical practice in their specialty. Their practice
sessions last for six or seven hours a day, or even
longer. They begin long before the sun rises and
continue long after it sets, following this schedule
for years at a time. But they have a clear idea of
what they want to achieve, what goals they seek to
accomplish—they strive to be the fittest person in
their field, the one who can win the prize.

Paul says that these principles of training work for
the spiritual life, too. He says, "I do not run like a
man running aimlessly; I do not fight like a man
beating the air. No, I beat my body and make it my
slave so that after I have preached to others, I
myself will not be disqualified for the prize'' (1 Corinthians 9:26, 27). Paul says that he wants to be the
best witness for God he can possibly be. God made
him that, and more—a towering figure in the history
of Christianity.

Very few of us can be Olympic athletes setting

new records, important historical figures, or spiritual giants. But we can be the best and fittest persons, physically, mentally, and spiritually, that we are capable of being. To accomplish this we must have a commitment to begin our training, with a goal in sight. What is your prize? What will lure you to be "less" than you should be or more than you are? What weighs you down now from following this pattern of fitness?

Do you have a picture in your mind of what it would be like to be fit? Several years ago I couldn't imagine it. So when I began my journey to fitness and discipline, I simply trusted that God would provide me with that mental picture. It took a while to emerge, but I was patient.

As I shared my struggle with some of my ministerial colleagues, an individual minister took time to tell me what had happened to him. He had lost forty pounds over a period of time when he had begun the same workout plan I had followed. He encouraged me, told me of his success in maintaining his weight, and, most importantly, he prayed with me. I could unburden my soul to him, and he would understand. How rarely this level of sharing occurs between ministers, between men—between many Christians in our churches.

You must ask for prayerful support from friends as you begin your program so that you receive encouragement as you gradually become the fit person you want to be. Since losing my weight and meeting my goals I have tried to take up this ministry of encouragement to others. That is one of the reasons why I have written this book.

As one of my goals I determined to run and finish a 6.2 mile race. I trained carefully and built up my speed and endurance. I had no idea of how much time I would take to finish, and I told myself again and again that I was not competing against *anyone* else, only myself; I was testing the level of fitness I had achieved. I had been running steadily for only four months when I set the run before me.

Running—or any competitive athletic activity— was something I had never imagined myself attempting. When I was in high school, I had two distinguished records in physical education. One was for the *longest* time ever recorded by a student in the mile-run. That takes tremendous exertion! The other was for the *shortest* career on the school gymnastics team. I must have had a lot of gall to join the team in the shape I was in. My specialty was—get this— the *trampoline*. What a sight I must have been, all 200 pounds hurtling through space attempting somersaults, defying laws of gravity and honor. Extra spotters always managed to appear as I began my bounce—whether for further protection or greater amusement, I was never sure. I lasted one week. The coach let me keep my dignity—he allowed me to resign from the team.

So as a result I didn't have a very successful image of training. This time, however, training was going much better, and I became increasingly excited as the day of the run came closer. I could feel the wellness and fitness surging through my body; the only other times I have run like that have been in preparation for other "races": the day of my wedding and the day before the birth of my first child.

The day of the race came, and I was prepared. I had had a good night's sleep. The night before I had actually eaten some of my favorite forbiddens—lasagna, bread, cheesecake (this last one was a special treat, not on the John Throop Official Training Diet). I ate lightly that morning and walked to the starting line, about one-half mile away. I warmed up carefully, ran several paces, met other runners, and fell somewhere into the middle of the human mass—with over two thousand other runners. I prayed quietly for endurance and strength, focused my mind on the run route, and prayed some more.

It may not have been the Olympics, but it might as well have been for me. The starting gun went off, and I bolted forward. I ran, and ran well, feeling good throughout the race, pouring on "the gas" at the end, seeing nothing in sight but the finish line. I crossed the line to cheers, to smiling parishioners, and to great news—I placed in the top half with a time of forty-four minutes—a seven-and-a-half-minute mile! Amazing!

A couple of years later I ran another race and placed in the top quarter! Training for races, if you are a runner—or for some event in your own sport—helps to focus the goal for fitness and call out the commitment. You often excel at what you thought you could never do.

So as you discipline yourself for fitness, you must believe that anything is possible, with God's help. That's why you must attend not only to your physical fitness or mental discipline, but your spiritual fitness as well. Those deep spiritual wells are your source of power.

A final key to fitness is *consistency,* a brother to balance and discipline. Seek to be consistent in your fitness; be regular about your routine. Your power for consistency will originate in your spiritual life— your discipline in having some quiet time to listen to the Lord God, to read his Word, to pray for your own needs and those of others. If you can be consistent in your spiritual life, you should be able to find consistency in what you eat and how you exercise.

A friend of mine is a self-professed weekend athlete. He has a stressful job which requires him to work with troubled people. For most of his day he is inactive physically. But on weekends, look out! He likes to play softball, tennis, and racquetball, and he enjoys skiing during the winter months. But he has no regular plan of exercise, is somewhat overweight and definitely poorly conditioned. He does not even engage in his preferred sports with consistency. Then he wonders why he pulls muscles or twists joints.

If he were consistent even on weekends, and did just a little bit of conditioning every day, he would be able to avoid injury. He probably would manage to avoid a coronary. If you set out a plan for exercise, *do it.* If you miss a day, or even two days, *don't overexercise to make up for what you've lost.* This principle is especially important if you miss for weeks at a time—for instance, if you have had the flu, with residual weakness.

Likewise, if you eat an item which really is to be avoided on a careful eating program, don't starve yourself in reaction the next day. As time passes, you should have developed a pattern of eating and exercise which is consistent enough to allow an occasional lapse. But if your experience is anything like mine, you will *want* to exercise and you'll miss it when you can't do it. You will want to eat healthful foods because you feel terrible after eating that rich dessert—and I mean more than emotionally so.

Consistency, balance, and discipline should be the hallmarks of a Christian's approach to life in general, and to the use of the body and its fitness in particular. In a word, these three are dimensions of *self-control*, a fruit of the Spirit of God. God is the source of self-control. God is the beginning and end of all our efforts toward fitness. We are fit Christians in order to glorify God.

The principles which make for a sound spiritual and mental life also make for a sound physical life—they are all part of that marvelous package called the human body, the human *being*. We are stewards of that body God has given us. God helps us to use this body wisely. He gives us the power to be fit Christians, not fat Christians.

Let's stop letting our bodies grow like so much suburban sprawl, with no plan for development, resulting only in clogged arteries. Let's think through carefully the kind of *human beings in bodies* that we want to be, that God wants us to be. Let us not run aimlessly nor box at the air, but let us instead develop a plan to become the disciplined, happy, healthy people we were meant to be.

God gave us the potential for fitness, so let us follow his plans, not seeking to add on to his blueprints for our bodies. It is our responsibility to eat and exercise with care, and to educate ourselves about the principles of fitness. It is our task to shape up—from the inside out.

Be patient and pray for endurance as you set out on your journey to fitness. It is an exciting journey to health and real contentment because you feel *well*. God wants it for you; you have to want it for yourself to become fit. You have only your weight to lose—and your life to gain!

EPILOGUE

The diet had worked. The exercise seemingly was effortless, and I felt like a million dollars. I was down to 163 pounds, decked out in a new summer-weight suit (after having donated my corpulent-size clothes—many of them still very new—to the Salvation Army). Members of the congregation queried me. Yes, I felt fine—better than I ever had felt. No, I wasn't feeling weak. No, I wasn't going to lose any more. No, it wasn't easy. And so on.

About that time, the movie *Chariots of Fire* made its first run. Seeing the movie was a very emotional experience for me—in my own small way, I felt like Eric Liddell, the runner with spiritual and physical discipline. I was inspired!

Those scenes of running on the beach got to me. I grew up on the shores of Lake Michigan near sand and water. I had given my life over to Christ while walking on a beach in California. Beaches are very special, relaxing, healing, celebrating places for me.

I had a birthday coming, and I decided to give myself a gift: a trip to Bermuda, with its fabled pink

beaches and laid-back family atmosphere. I would go alone to think about and pray over the course of my life in the next few years. I was a different person than I had ever been before—a healthy, vigorous, athletic person. What would God do with my life now?

I went, and had the most glorious vacation ever— a time of rest, sun, good solitude, and great bike riding up and down the hills. I grew very tan and even a little thinner with the cycling I did through the island. I returned to Chicago and my prayer partner minister picked me up at the airport. He told me how rested and fit I looked.

Early that week I went to my denomination's regional office in downtown Chicago to chair the first meeting of a new committee. As I stepped into the elevator to go to the meeting room, a woman entered to attend the same meeting, and we struck up a conversation. She met the new John Throop.

We married a year later.

Sometimes fitness really pays off.